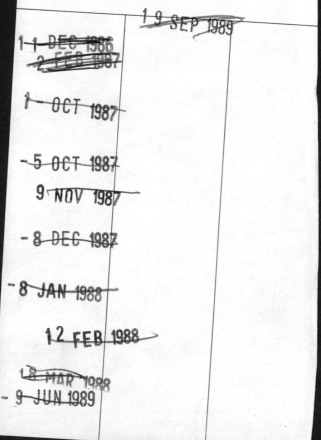

MEDICAL BOOK
ILLUSTRATION

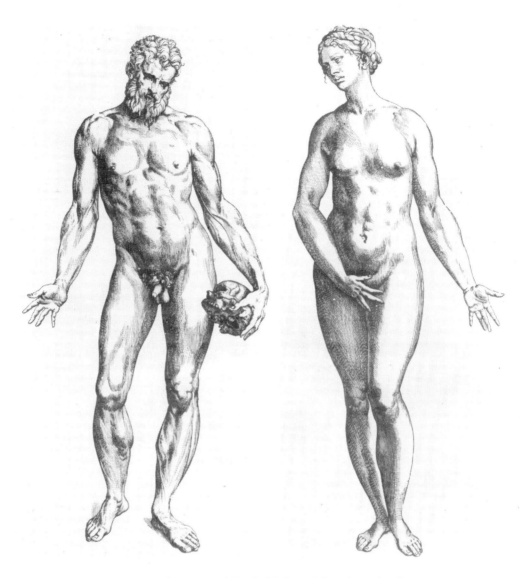

Frontispiece. "Adam and Eve". Male and female nudes from
Andreas Vesalius' *Epitome*, [1543].

MEDICAL BOOK ILLUSTRATION

A short history

JOHN L. THORNTON F.L.A.

Formerly
Librarian, St. Bartholomew's Hospital
Medical College

Consulting Librarian, Royal College of Obstetricians
and Gynaecologists

and

CAROLE REEVES, A.I.I.P.

Senior Medical Photographer
Institute of Child Health and
Hospital for Sick Children, Great Ormond Street,
London

THE OLEANDER PRESS
Cambridge   New York
1983

The Oleander Press
17 Stansgate Avenue
Cambridge CB2 2QZ
England

The Oleander Press
210 Fifth Avenue
New York
N.Y. 10010
U.S.A.

First published 1983

M7258

14/3/83

British Library Cataloguing in Publication Data
Thornton, John Leonard
    Medical book illustration.—(Oleander medical
book series; v. 2)
    1. Medical illustration
    I. Title
    600.2'42   R836

    ISBN 0-906672-07-4

Designed by Graham Taverner
Set in 12pt Plantin by Alphaset Typesetting, Cambridge
Printed and bound in Great Britain

☙ CONTENTS ☙

TO THE MEMORY OF
VERA THORNTON
(1915-1982)

≋ LIST OF ILLUSTRATIONS ≋

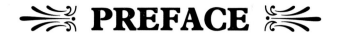

PREFACE

This book is intended as an introduction to the history of medical book illustration, and in a short "helicopter flight" over the subject we can only view the highlights, descending at intervals to examine specimens of outstanding examples in each period. We have concentrated mainly on the activities of artists and engravers in illustrating medical texts, and have only touched upon medical photography and other mechanical aids as ancillary to medical art. They require treatment in a separate volume.

For teaching purposes, illustrations can be more informative than pages of written matter, and many books have survived as items of interest and information solely on the importance and value of the work of the artists involved. Their work can have a practical application in the teaching of medical students and artists. The recent dramatic increase in the use of audio-visual aids and in the number of departments devoted to the subject in teaching institutions has created new interest in the visual aids of the past, and the artists creating them can be emulated to advantage.

The illustrations are reproduced from various sources, the originals often being very much larger than the reproductions. To appreciate their full significance one must see the original volumes, where the texture of the paper, the technology of the printer, engraver and colourist reveal the full beauty of the endeavours of the artist. As black-and-white miniatures of the original plates they serve only to illustrate the text, and to prompt the interested reader to consult the originals when possible.

We are grateful to the staffs of the following libraries who have been particularly helpful in providing information and supplying photocopies: the Wellcome Institute for the History of Medicine; the Royal College of Obstetricians and Gynaecologists; the Royal College of Surgeons of England; the Institute of Child Health and the Hospital for Sick Children, Great Ormond Street, Department of Medical Illustration; and St. Thomas's Hospital Medical School. Numerous individuals have also supplied information and material, including Mr. William R. LeFanu, Mr. Peter Cull, Dr. Robert Ollerenshaw, Dr. Clifford Shepley, Cynthia Clarke, Susan White and

Margaret McLarty. We also wish to thank the copyright holders, who are named in the captions, for permission to reproduce the illustrations. Mrs. Ann Munson typed the manuscript, and we are very grateful to her for her skilful interpretation of a difficult manuscript.

June 1982   J.L.T.
                                                                                               C.R.

⇒ CHAPTER 1 ⇐

MATERIALS, METHODS AND GENERAL SOURCES

"The figuration of the anatomic form of man by the graphic arts aims either to make the teaching of human anatomy more plastic for the anatomist and physiologist, engraving it on the memory, or to give the plastic artist a clear, scientific basis for his studies of the human figure".

Ludwig Choulant; translated by Mortimer Frank.

The history of the development of medical book illustration has obviously been governed by the materials and techniques available. Drawings on cave walls, stone inscriptions, and the carving of models from bone or stone were followed by inscriptions on bamboo, silk, papyrus, parchment and paper, executed with a pen or brush. Wet clay in tablet form was incised by means of a stylus, but although pictograms and hieroglyphics depicted human subjects, very few strictly medical subjects were represented.

The book as we know it was preceded by the roll or folded sheet of material, and even a stack of clay tablets, being a record of events, might be termed a "book" despite the fact that the leaves would be of clay. The development of the codex form, with folded leaves, and with covers or bindings, made the book both easier to handle and to store. It also facilitated the task of the scribe and the illuminator, but the invention of printing, particularly from movable type, promoted the rapid growth of literature of all types. Initially the illustrations were confined to woodcuts, since these could be printed with the text, but these were soon followed by engravings and the products of other methods of reproduction, as outlined below.

There are three basic methods of printing illustrations: relief, where the design is printed in relief, the background being cut away; intaglio, in which the design is incised on a block or plate, which is inked and the surface is wiped clean, strong pressure forcing the paper into the incisions, the result showing a "plate-line", although this is often trimmed by the binder; and planograph, where the design is drawn on a flat surface, printing being effected by using ink-resistant material where the plate is to remain clear of ink.

Woodcuts were in use at an early date in the Far East, and first appeared in Europe soon after 1400. In block-books, text and figures were cut upon the same piece of wood, and were therefore printed together. With the invention of movable type, woodcuts could still be placed side by side with the text and printed simultaneously. Towards the end of the fifteenth century soft metal was sometimes used instead of wood, but metalcuts do not have so sharp-edged an effect. They never, of course, develop cracks or worm-holes, which are often noticed in woodcuts used over a period of years.

15

Wood-engravings are distinguished from woodcuts by the predominance of white lines, and are cut on the end grain of hard woods, such as box, pear or yew, with a graver or gouge instead of a knife. This process was made popular by the outstanding work of Thomas Bewick (1753-1828). Unfortunately for our purpose, he was mainly concerned with the depiction of natural history subjects, and no medical prints by him have been noted. Wood engraving was ousted by the popularity of other media, but was again widely used in the nineteenth century, and even used in an attempt to reproduce photographs. However, when "half-tone" and other methods were introduced, it was reserved for its original purpose, and is still employed to great advantage. Lino-cuts, which give a coarser appearance, were a recent development, the blocks consisting of linoleum.

Engraving on metal by means of a burin, which acts like a plough, followed upon woodcuts as the most popular method of book illustration. Copper was the material most commonly employed, probably because, being soft, lines were more easily incised. However, this also resulted in a limit to the number of crisp copies which could be printed, and later, steel was introduced, or the copper plates were coated with this material. Plates had to be printed separately from the text, as in other processes of engraving, since the actual printed surface was the result of paper being forced into the depressions made by the engraver. The resultant plates were either inserted between the normally printed pages, or grouped together at the end of the volume. A useful feature was introduced whereby folding plates were printed a page width from the spine of the book. When unfolded the plates could readily be consulted in conjunction with the appropriate pages of the text. A few examples of copper engraving are found in fifteenth-century books.

Mezzotint was a method of copper engraving in which the plate was first roughened all over by means of a "rocker", or fine metal-toothed comb. Highlights and half-tones were obtained by scraping away the burr with a knife, and polishing with a burnisher. Attempts were made at using different coloured inks on separate plates, but this process was little used for the reproduction of medical subjects. Examples are mentioned in Chapter 5. The process was invented in Germany about 1642 by Ludwig van Siegen, and was brought by Prince Rupert to England, where it became popular in the reproduction of portraits and oil paintings.

Etching is a form of engraving in which acid is used to eat into a copper plate which has been coated with a varnish or with resin. The copper is evenly coated with powdered resin and gently heated so that it sticks to the plate, or the resin is dissolved in alcohol before application; a needle or similar implement is used as a pencil to remove the resin and, when the acid is applied to the plate, it eats into the metal. The depth is controlled by stopping with varnish between exposures to the acid, and etched and engraved plates are printed by the same technique. Sometimes the processes are combined in one plate. It will be obvious that the artist has closely to supervise the preparation of the plates, taking samples at intervals to ensure that the finished plate meets his requirements. The plates also have to be printed separately from the text.

Aquatint, a variety of etching, possibly first used about 1650, was rarely employed until a century later, when it is commonly said to have been invented by Jean Baptiste Le Prince about 1768. When acid is applied to the plate a fine network of lines is etched on the surface, giving a granular effect, which when printed gives a tone similar to water-colour wash. Aquatint is generally used in conjunction with etching. In dry-point etching the incisions are made directly into the copper without acid being employed. These processes and their numerous variations in technique are fully described by E.S. Lumsden (1962) in *The art of etching*, which provides full information on the tools employed, methods and materials, and is illustrated with 152 plates.

Lithography was discovered in 1796 by Alois Senefelder (1771-1834), and thus produced the planograph, or flat-bed printing. Many improvements both in material and technique were introduced subsequently, but originally a drawing was made with greasy ink or chalk on a kind of limestone which is porous to grease and water. The stone was then damped with water, and a roller loaded with greasy ink was passed over it. Paper was then laid on the stone, the whole being passed through a scraper press. The resultant impression shows subtle gradations of tone.

Written as a guide to scientists in selecting the best process available for use to illustrate their writings, *The essentials of illustration* by T.G. Hill (1915) provides technical details of the various processes. It suggests the best techniques, and gives examples of each. The author also includes some identical illustrations reproduced by different techniques, to emphasize the advantages of certain processes for particular purposes. A more general survey of the subject was made by R. Margaret Slythe (1970) in *The art of illustration, 1750-1900*, which has chapters devoted to the woodcut and the wood-engraving; the etching; the engraving; and the lithograph.

The most significant book in the history of medical illustration is without doubt *History and bibliography of anatomic illustration* by Ludwig Choulant (1945). Originally published in 1852, the German version was translated into English by Mortimer Frank, who added considerable supplementary material. Subsequent editions contain additional essays, and the work is a monumental contribution to the subject. Well illustrated, it contains full bibliographical details of the items cited, with biographical information on the authors and artists. Unfortunately, even the 1962 reprint is not readily available.

Other useful books with an emphasis on medical illustration include *Storia dell' iconografia anatomica*, by Loris Premuda (1956); *Geschichte der gynäkologisch-anatomischen Abbildungen*, by Fritz Weindler (1908), which is arranged on a similar plan to Choulant, but surpasses that work in the variety of its illustrations, and obviously has emphasis on gynaecological material; Robert Herrlinger's *Geschichte der medizinischen Abbildung*, second edition 1967, was translated into English by Graham Fulton-Smith as *History of medical illustration from antiquity to A.D. 1600*, 1970. This was followed by a second volume in German by Marielene Putscher (1972) with the title *Geschichte der medizinischen Abbildung. Von 1600 bis zur Gegenwart*. These cover all types of medical illustration, and are well illustrated, some of the plates being in colour.

Although based on the collection in one particular library, *Histoire de la médecine et du livre médical, à la lumière des collections de la Bibliothèque de la Faculté de Médecine de Paris*, by André Hahn and others (1962), is a valuable contribution to the history of medical illustration. The numerous illustrations, some in colour, are supported by an authoritative text, and reveal something of the richness of the library at the Faculté de Médecine in Paris. Another book containing numerous plates, and based on a collection of medical books, is *Notable medical books from the Lilly Library, Indiana University*, compiled by William R. LeFanu (1976). This beautifully-produced volume contains descriptions of 130 of the most important medical books contained in the collection, and most of the illustrations are of plates in these items. The texts facing the plates often provide information on the artists and processes involved. William LeFanu (1972) has also contributed an interesting article on some English illustrated books, which contain six plates.

An interesting address on the history of art in its relation to medical science was published by William Anderson (1886), which surveys the scene from antiquity to the nineteenth century. Well illustrated with plates from outstanding medical books, it also briefly mentions paintings, sculpture, and models in wax as examples of art in medicine. Other general articles dealing with illustrations in printed medical books include contributions by C.P. Rollins (1949); Ruth B. Coleman (1950), writing on the illustration of human anatomy before Vesalius; J. Whillis (1951) on anatomical illustrations; Helmuth M. Nathan (1976) on art in medicine; and Louis G. Audette (1979) contributed an interesting article on stylism in anatomical illustration from the sixteenth to the eighteenth centuries, to show the effects of advances in methods of reproduction and printing.

A brief history of medical illustration was published by William E. Loechel (1960), and a more extensive survey by Thomas S. Jones (1959) brought the subject up to the time of writing. T.S. Jones was at one time Professor of Medical and Dental Illustrations at the University of Illinois College of Medicine, Chicago. Himself an outstanding medical artist, he was responsible for training many others in the subject.

A more general volume on illustrated books has recently been written by John Harthan (1981) as *The history of the illustrated book. The western tradition*. This is profusely illustrated with 465 plates, several of them being in colour. It covers the subject chronologically from the Egyptian and Byzantine periods, and brings the subject up to date in a sumptuously-produced volume which is a model of book production at its best. It is completed by a useful section containing notes on techniques, and an extensive list of references.

⚛ CHAPTER 2 ⚛

ANCIENT MEDICAL ILLUSTRATION

"The sources of our knowledge lie in what is written on bamboo and silk, what is engraved on metal and stone, and what is cut on vessels to be handed down to posterity."

Mo Tzu, 5th century B.C.

Although this book is concerned with medical book illustration, we must remember that the codex form was not that initially used for medical texts, and that the illustration of medical subjects was not confined to manuscripts written on papyrus, parchment, paper or similar materials. Jürgen Thorwald (1962) in *Science and secrets of early medicine* covers Egypt, Mesopotamia, India, China, Mexico and Peru in a well-illustrated history, with an excellent bibliography but, for obvious reasons, few of the illustrations are from books. They are examples of art in medicine, and medicine in art, and must be considered as overlapping the periods in which illustrations were used to elucidate the text.

Ancient Egypt has provided us with abundant material relating to the history of medicine in the form of papyri, mummies, inscriptions and wall-paintings, and Carole Reeves (1980) has provided a study of the subject containing figures illustrating the various techniques and materials employed. Around 200 A.D. the founder of a Christian school in Alexandria, Flavius Clemens, recorded that before the beginning of the Old Kingdom period (2780-2280 B.C.), the priests had collected all knowledge into forty-two secret, sacred books. Among these were six books dealing with anatomy, physiology, surgery, pharmacology and female ailments. The original source of all the medical papyri are these six books mentioned by Flavius Clemens. The sacred books are known as the Hermetic books because they were ascribed to the God Thoth, whom the Greeks named Hermes Trismegistos. They were kept as sacred in the temples, and the priests of the highest of the eight castes of the priesthood studied all forty-two of them. The pastophores, the members of the lowest caste, studied only the six medical books.

In 1873, a German Egyptologist, Georg Ebers, acquired in Thebes a papyrus scroll which had been discovered in a tomb about 1860 (Plate 1). Originally it was a roll sixty-eight feet long, but divided into pages of twenty lines each, totalling 108 columns, the scribe wrongly numbering them 110. The roll was cut up and bound in modern form, and is now housed in the University Library at Leipzig. On the reverse are calendar notations which date its origin as about 1555 B.C. It contains 876 remedies, and mentions 500 substances used in

19

medical treatment. It also contains a considerable amount of magico-religious therapy, as well as notes on eye diseases and surgery. Trachoma, which is still known as Egyptian eye disease, and remains the chief cause of blindness in the East, is also mentioned. Concern with eye ailments and their prevention was one reason why the Egyptians wore heavy eye make-up, which served both as a salve and decoration. The Ebers Papyrus also contains fifty-five prescriptions in which faeces and urine are the main components. A facsimile edition of the papyrus was published by Ebers in two volumes in 1875; Walter Wreszinski published a hieroglyphic transcript in 1913; Bendix Ebbell published an English translation in 1937; and in 1957 Hermann Grapow, Hildegard von Deines and Wolfhart Westendorf published a more comprehensive translation of the Papyrus Ebers.

Edwin Smith, an American Egyptologist, bought a papyrus roll in Luxor in 1862 (Plate 1). It was fifteen feet, four inches long, and thirteen inches wide. On one side there are seventeen columns, each consisting of seventy-seven lines, and the reverse has four-and-a-half columns of ninety-two lines each. It has been dated at about 1600 B.C., but Old Kingdom words used in the text suggest that the papyrus was in fact copied from a work written around 2500 B.C. In 1930 James Henry Breasted published in two volumes a facsimile and hieroglyphic transliteration, with a translation and commentary, and the papyrus is now in the New York Academy of Medicine. The Edwin Smith Papyrus contains descriptions of forty-eight surgical cases, mostly traumatic in origin. There are sixty-nine appendices which explained to readers of 1600 B.C. certain expressions used in the original earlier language. The reverse side of the papyrus contains magical incantations and prescriptions. It is of particular interest because it contains the first description of the brain, observed in patients with extensive head wounds. The Egyptians recognised the fact that patients exhibiting such skull damage as to expose the brain and enable the surface to be described were beyond the scope of their healing powers.

The Hearst Papyrus, dating from about 1550 B.C., appears to be the formulary of a practising physician. It is incomplete, and contains eighteen columns. The hieratic text was published with a vocabulary by George A. Reisner in 1905, and a transliteration and German translation by Walter Wreszinski of this and the London Papyrus, dated about 1350 B.C. was published together in 1912. The Hearst Papyrus is preserved in the University of California, and the London Papyrus is in the British Museum.

During the course of excavations at Sakkara, Heinrich Brugsch found a jar containing a papyrus. This has been dated around 1350-1200 B.C., and contains 279 lines of prescriptions. The Berlin Medical Papyrus, dating from about 1300 B.C., contains about two hundred prescriptions, and both were described and translated by Walter Wreszinski in 1909. The Chester Beatty Papyrus in the British Museum was written about 1200 B.C., and deals with diseases of the anus. It contains eight columns, and is incomplete. A French translation, with annotations by F. Jonckheere, was published in 1947.

In 1898 Sir Flinders Petrie discovered during his excavations at Kahun a papyrus variously dated between 2100 and 1900 B.C. It consists of only three

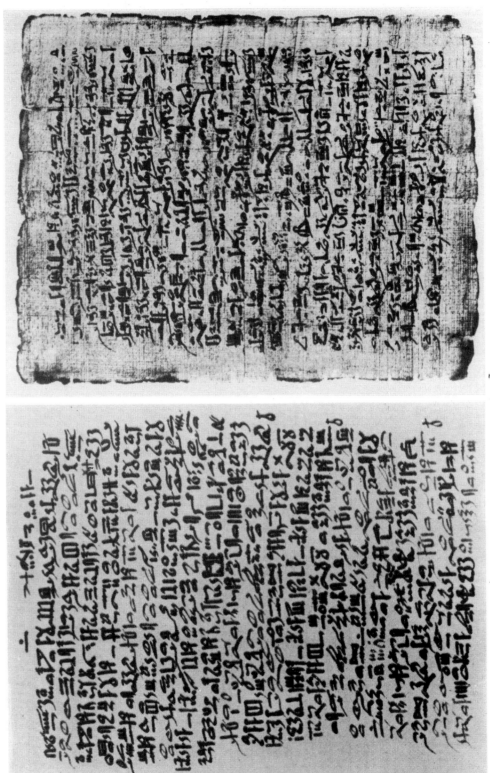

Plate 1. Sections from the Papyrus Ebers (left), and from the Edwin Smith Papyrus (right).

pages, and is preserved at University College, London. Devoted to diseases of women and pregnancy, it was published as a hieratic transcript with a translation by Francis Llewelyn Griffith in 1898, and is possibly the oldest medical papyrus to be discovered.

Both the Edwin Smith Papyrus and the Ebers Papyrus mention the heart, its beating, and the pulses to be found in the extremeties. The Egyptians conceived the idea of there being channels throughout the body carrying air, blood, semen, nourishment and waste, and not unnaturally likened this idea of a life flow to the flow and annual inundations of the Nile, upon which they depended for their very existence. The Veterinary Papyrus is the only papyrus written entirely in hieroglyphs, all the others being in the hieratic script, which is a simplified form of the hieroglyph. The only illustrated papyrus is the Papyrus of Ani, dating from about 1250 B.C., containing the Book of the Dead.

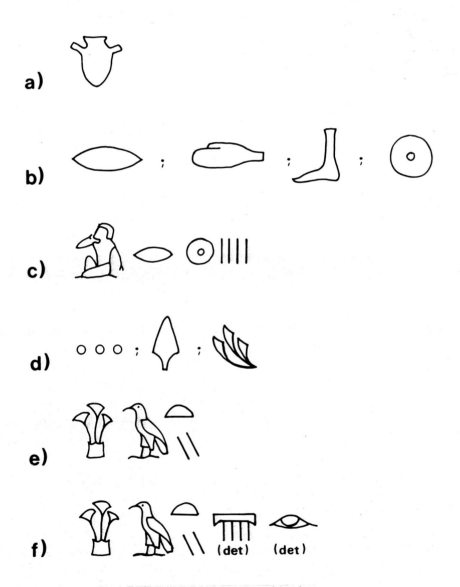

Plate 2. Hieroglyphics mentioned in the text.

In many instances the translation of the script on papyri is made easier by the fact that many of the hieroglyphs and hieratic writings are readily identifiable as pictograms. For example, the hieroglyph on Plate 2, Figure a, means "heart", and is a stylized form of the actual organ. Similarly, the pictograms on Plate 2, Figure b, meaning "mouth", "hand", "foot", and "sun", can fairly easily be identified. The prescription (Plate 2, Figure c) means 'take by mouth four times a day.' However, this was a spoken language and all hieroglyphs had sounds, so that very often the pictograms were used phonetically, and stood not for the objects themselves but for the sound used to make up part of the whole word. Nevertheless, the Egyptians did use illustrations in their writings to represent anatomical features.

A drawback to translating Egyptian hieroglyphs lies in the fact that they represent consonants, or groups of consonants, with no vowels, so that many unrelated words could have the same appearance when set down in pictographic form. The Egyptians avoided this by using a determinative at the end of a word to convey its sense. These determinatives, numbering about one hundred in common use, have proved invaluable in aiding our understanding and translating prescriptions and descriptions of illnesses which may have no equivalent in modern language. For example, many drugs and medicines used in Egypt would be unrecognizable without the necessary determinatives to identify the root source. Thus the determinatives on Plate 2, Figure d, following the drug names, tell us that they were respectively either of mineral, plant or herbal origin. Similarly, an unknown disease depicted on Plate 2, Figure e, and transliterated as "haty", would be meaningless without the determinative hieroglyphs on Plate 2, figure f. These represent rain falling from a cloud on an eye, so that we have a clear idea what sort of disease "haty" in fact was. (See Breasted, J.H., 1950; Hurry, J.B., 1928; and Mertz, Barbara, 1964).

The fact that the roots of Mesopotamian medicine reached back to the third millennium B.C. can be proved by the discovery in the 1890s of what is considered to be one of the earliest known medical "handbooks" carved on a clay tablet 3¾ inches by 6¼ inches in cuneiform script and bearing a collection of prescriptions (Plate 3). It was translated in 1952 by Samuel Noah Kramer and Martin Levey. The Land of the Two Rivers was the name given in the second century B.C. by the Greek historian Polybius to the region between the Tigris and the Euphrates. The first settlers in this area in the fourth millennium B.C. were the Sumerians. Around 2350 B.C. the Semitic warriors to the north and east of Mesopotamia invaded the fertile Sumerian valleys and, initially under Sargon of Akkad, ruled for two hundred years. The Sumerians then regained power until 1955 B.C., when Semitic tribes entered the Land of the Two Rivers. One of these tribal rulers was King Hammurabi (1728-1686 B.C.), who created an empire around the city of Babylon, and set down a list of laws known as the Code of Hammurabi. Of the 282 laws, nine are devoted to procedures for the practice of medicine. Among these are set out correct charges for treatment, punishments for malpractice, and the first reference to the operation of couching for cataract.

As the empire around Babylon developed, the temptation to subjugate its

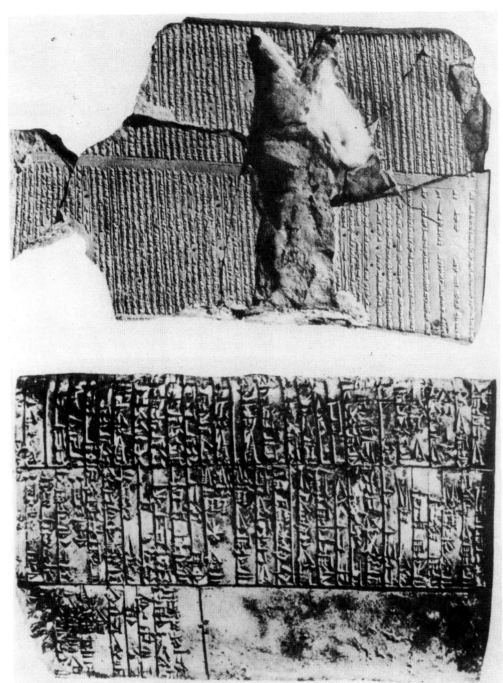

Plate 3. Medical clay tablets. Sumerian, third millennium B.C. (left). From the Library of King Assurbanipal, Mesopotamia (right).

people and to share its riches became irresistible to the warlords of Assyria, and in about 1100 B.C. King Tiglathpileser I of Assyria became the first of a long line of warrior-rulers. The most notorious of these was Assurbanipal (Ashurbanipal) (668-626 B.C.) who hung the flayed skins of his enemies from the walls of their conquered cities. Despite his barbarity, King Assurbanipal collected together an extensive library at Kouyunjik, which was excavated by Sir Henry Layard. He discovered about 30,000 fragments of cuneiform clay tablets, 606 of which contain medical texts (Plate 3). These are all in the British Museum, and facsimiles and translations of the medical texts have been published by Reginald Campbell Thompson (1923 and 1924-26).

Towards the end of the nineteenth century an American archaeological team unearthed a large library at the Sumerian city of Nippur, where the earliest known clay prescription was found, discovering a set of physicians' reports dating from about 2000 B.C. which deal with the health and well-being of the female members of an establishment for singers and dancers. In the mountainous area of Anatolia, several hundred miles to the north of Mesopotamia, the Hittite Empire arose during the second millennium B.C. In the 1950s its capital city of Hattusas was excavated, and many clay tablets of medical texts were discovered. They are particularly interesting because they are Hittite copies of earlier Mesopotamian texts.

In addition to medical prescriptions and descriptions of plagues and diseases, the Land of the Two Rivers also yielded the oldest known letters of early physicians. The Tigris-Euphrates Valley was rife with bubonic and pneumonic plagues and malaria, to which Alexander the Great succumbed in Babylon in 324 B.C. Descriptions of plagues and fevers are prevalent in many of the medical texts from the earliest Mesopotamian finds through to the Old Testament, notably in the First Book of Samuel, which records the traumatic conflicts between the Philistines and Israelites in the eleventh century B.C.

Reginald Campbell Thompson, in addition to his writings on Assyrian medical texts (Thompson, 1923; 1924-6), was also the author of *The Assyrian herbal*, 1924, a compilation of 250 named drugs, plants, minerals and herbs in medicinal use, the clinical trials of which were performed on slaves and prisoners.

The Aryan conquerors who moved into the Indus Valley from the north-west in the middle of the second millennium B.C., the Hindus, provide us with the earliest surviving writings of Ancient India. The famous collections of verse, the Vedas, comprise the Samaveda (the Art of Melody), the Rigveda (the Art of Hymns), the Atharvaveda (the Art of Charms and Incantations), and the Ayurveda (the Art of Life). They record something of the cultures and politics of these early settlers, and the Ayurveda is the most important as far as medicine is concerned. From this early Indian culture arose two important religio-intellectual movements, Jainism and Buddhism.

The fierce dissension within the existing caste system paved the way for the invasion by Alexander the Great in 326 B.C. Upon his death in Babylon two years later, Seleucus I attempted to re-occupy the Punjab, but was thwarted by King Chandragupta Maurya of Magadhu, creator of the Maurya Empire which was to unite most of India for the next one hundred and fifty years. King Asoka of the Maurya Empire (273-232 B.C) became a convert to Buddhism, and was a great patron of the arts and sciences. Upon his death, the Mauryan Empire collapsed, and India again became disunited. Buddhism and Hinduism remained forever split.

In 997 A.D., Islamic armies from Afghanistan entered India, to add yet another culture. The Ayurveda, a supplement to the Atharvaveda, contains the first references to medicine and medical practice in India after the Aryan invasion, and endemic diseases can readily be identified. The symptoms of typhoid, leprosy, smallpox, cholera and many other diseases can be recognized in the text. Magic and ritual and the idea of sin's being the cause of disease and illness were fundamental to Indian medical lore, but the importance of drug use was also stressed. The Rigveda mentions the manufacture of prosthetic limbs, and the removal of injured eyes, most amputations being necessitated by the traumatic wounds of a fighting people. The city of Taxila in the north-west of India was the most important centre of medical learning in Ancient India, and one of the greatest in the Ancient World. The outstanding medical teacher, Atraya, to whom the origins of the Charaka Samhita are attributed, lived and worked in Taxila in the eighth or seventh century B.C. The Charaka Samhita (Plate 4) as a written text was not committed to manuscript until about 100 A.D., but its origins date back to Atraya, whose teachings are set out in the poetic style intended to be memorized and passed on by word of mouth. It is named after the physicians who wrote down the text.

Another important medical teaching centre in India was Benares, on the River Ganges, and its foremost teacher was Susruta, who was probably a contemporary of Atraya, and mentions him in his own teachings. The Susruta Samhita (Plate 4) although based on the teaching of Susruta, and named after him, was not written down until about 100 A.D., which makes it of contemporary textual origin with the Charaka Samhita. There is controversy over the date of the writing of the Susruta Samhita: Indian authorities have dated it within the first half of the first millennium B.C., but Western scholars have suggested the later date of about 100 A.D.

A Buddhist medical manuscript found in 1890 in Turkestan, and known as the Bower Manuscript after the English lieutenant who acquired it, was translated by the Sanskrit scholar Rudolf Hoernle between 1893 and 1897. Dating from the fifth century A.D., it mentions both the Charaka Samhita and the Susruta Samhita, specifically naming Charaka and Susruta as notable physicians. The Susruta Samhita is important because of its surgical content, and if its origins can indeed be dated back to the third or second millennium B.C., it has no rival in the Ancient World to compare with its surgical knowledge. Even if passages of later knowledge were subsequently added, it is still unique in its content, including a very fascinating passage describing in great detail the preparation of a corpse for dissection.

The Charaka Samhita was translated into Arabic and Persian in the tenth century A.D., and into Hindi, Gujarati and English in a six-volume work published by the Shree Gulabkunverba Ayurvedic Society in 1949. The Susruta

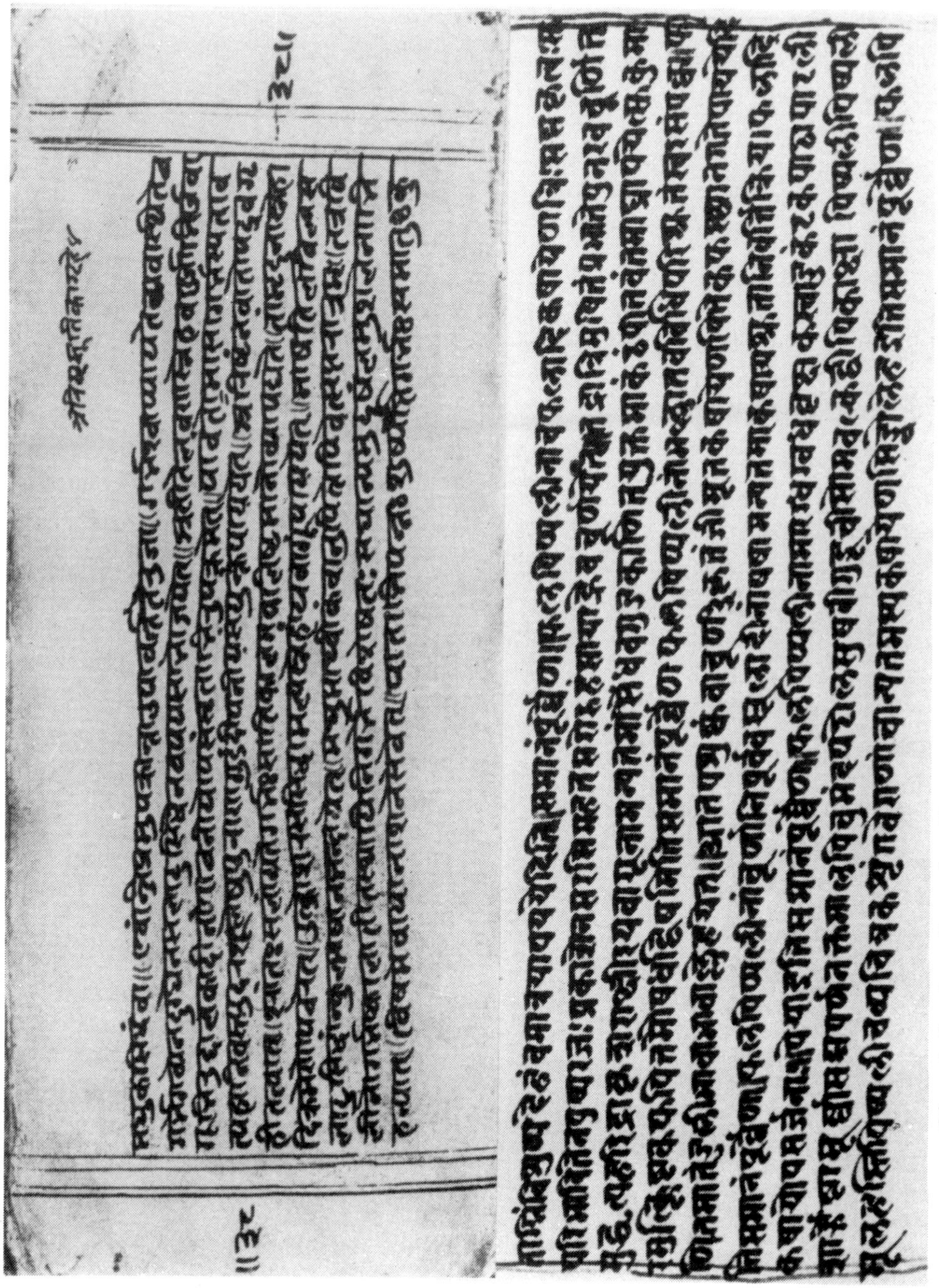

Plate 4. Sections from the *Charaka Samhita* (top), and the *Susruta Samhita* (bottom).

Samhita appeared in an English translation in two volumes published between 1907 and 1911. Unfortunately, neither of these two works is illustrated, and we have traced no Indian representations of medical subjects, apart from certain temple and similar carvings which appear to be anatomical without being strictly medical.

The beginnings of Chinese books and records have been the subject of a book by Tsuen-Hsuin Tsien (1962), in which he made a general survey of Chinese written records from about 1400 B.C. to about 700 A.D, when printing was being initiated. He covers records on bones and shells (particularly tortoise shells), inscriptions on metals and clay, engravings on stone and jade, and documents of bamboo and wood. Tsien describes silk as a writing material, the use of quasi-paper and paper in the production of manuscripts, and also deals with the tools and other materials used for writing.

The soil of Anyang, one-time capital of the Shang kings (1523-1028 B.C.), has yielded thousands of bones from the second millennium B.C. bearing inscriptions in characters not very different from the Chinese script of later periods. These inscriptions took the form of questions to the gods, and were later written on strips of bamboo. The Chou Empire (1027-256 B.C.) bequeathed to posterity four important books: "Shu Ching", the Book of History; "I Li", the Book of Ceremonies; "Shih Ching", the Book of Odes; and "I Ching", the Book of Prophecies. Under the Chou Empire, the land of China was distributed among one thousand knights, who founded their own principalities with a major city in each, and struggled amongst themselves to enlarge their own fiefs. Confucius (551-479 B.C.), the great philosopher, attempted to bring order to this chaotic Empire by preaching and practising virtue, simplicity and family order.

When Shih Huang Ti, the first acknowledged Emperor of China, came to power in 221 B.C., he ordered the destruction of all books except those dealing with agriculture, medicine and soothsaying. The "Shen Nung Pen Tsao" (Plate 5) was written down in the Chou period, and a late copy is to be found in a collection of drug recipes published in China in 1597 A.D, the *Pen Tshao Kang Mu*, or the Classification of Roots and Herbs (Plate 5). This collection, comprising fifty-two volumes, listed 1892 medicaments. Three hundred and sixty-five of the drugs dated from the Chou Empire.

Huang Ti (2698-2598 B.C.) is regarded as the father of the *Nei Chung*, purported to be the oldest medical publication in the world (Chen, 1969). The subjects are the functions of the human body, its diseases and their cure. The earliest versions of this book are accredited to writers of the Chou Empire, and it also deals in some detail with acupuncture. Medical writings dating from the Western Han Dynasty (206 B.C. — 8 A.D.), unearthed in Kansu Province, consist of thirty-five strips of wood bound together to form a book. They contain prescriptions, among which is one for the treatment of a horse.

Possibly the earliest comprehensive publication on the art of acupuncture was written during the Sung Dynasty by the eminent eleventh-century acupuncturist Wang Wei-I. This book, entitled *Tung Jen Ching*, was commissioned by the Emperor, who ordered Wang Wei-I to locate the meridian points of the human body for the sake of acupuncture practice. Printing reached a high

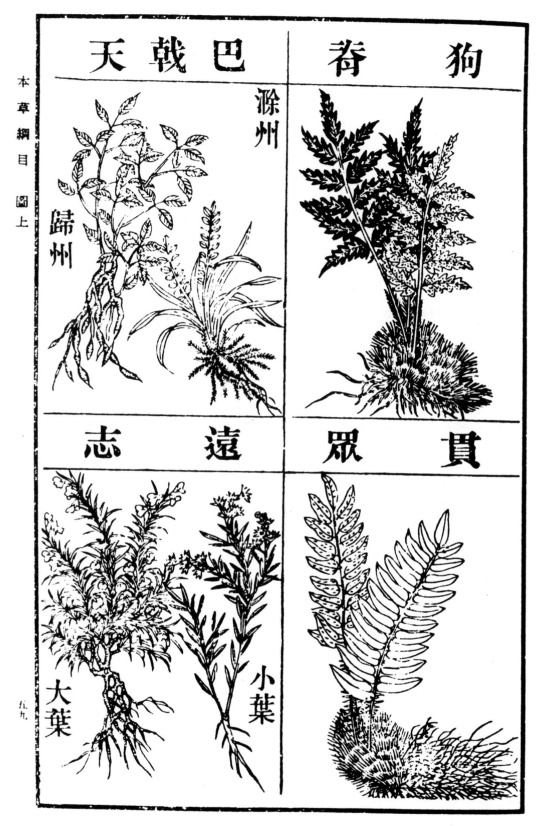

Plate 5. Pen Tshao Kang Mu, 1597. From a Chou Dynasty work, "Shen Nung Pen Tsao".
(1027-256 B.C.)

29

degree of perfection during the Sung Dynasty. The negatives were hand-carved on wooden plates, books printed from these being known as Sung-Press books.

It has been suggested that the first reported Chinese dissection was carried out on the body of a prisoner in 1145 A.D. (Thorwald, 1962), but the much later date of 1797 A.D. (Huard and Wong, 1959) would appear to be more acceptable, as early Chinese culture did not consider any form of dissection admissible. Early Chinese medicine was largely based on cosmology. The five major organs (heart, lung, liver, kidneys and spleen) were in constantly-fluctuating relationships of friendship and adversity with the five minor organs (the large intestine, the small intestine, gall bladder, stomach and bladder). The chief cause of all disease was a disturbance between Yin and Yang.

Dien Ch'io lived in the fifth or sixth century B.C., and is considered to be the originator of the *Nan Ching*, a work which tells us much about the methods of diagnosis, particularly on the Chinese observations of the pulse, which remained the key to the unlocking of internal maladies.

Hwa To (*c.* 190–265 A.D.) (Plate 6) was the first mentioned Chinese surgeon; he met an untimely end by offering to perform trepannation on a Chinese prince, Tsao Tsao, who was suffering unbearable headaches. The operation was never carried out as Tsao Tsao became suspicious of Hwa To, and ordered his execution. Hwa To asked that all his medical writings should be destroyed at the same time. As Hwa To had no successors for hundreds of years, it is possible that he was not of Chinese but of Asian origin, entering China through the Turkestan trade route to India. (See also Kan, Lai-Bing, 1965).

Medicine was introduced into Tibet from India in the seventeenth century, and the best source of information on Tibetan medicine is a book by the Ven. Rechung Rinpoche (1973). This contains a biography of the Great Physician-Saint gYu-thog the Elder (A.D. 786-911), who spread the knowledge of medicine throughout Tibet. It also includes translations of chapters from the second and fourth books of the "rGud-bzhi", a Sanskrit medical work written about A.D. 400, but which survives only in Tibetan and Mongolian translations. The book is illustrated with several Tibetan anatomical diagrams and two colour plates. They are mostly full-length figures indicating various venous systems, but also viscera, points for moxa, body measurements, and medical and surgical instruments.

We know that the various countries in South America reached high standards of civilization at an early age, but few written records of the period have survived. When in 1520 the Spanish Conquistadores marched into Tenochtitlán, it was the capital of the Aztec Empire. Until the coming of the Spaniards it was ruled by Montezuma II, and it was completely destroyed in the course of the ensuing battles. The Aztec Empire was breathtaking in its sophistication. The priests had a hieroglyphic form of writing which was evolving into a phonetic script. Paper was manufactured from the scraped bark of a genus of mulberry tree, or from the fibres of the wild fig tree. Great storehouses contained large numbers of documents, including records of legal proceedings, tribute lists and folded books. The Spaniards, in the name of religion and colonization, wreaked utter destruction upon the whole culture. A

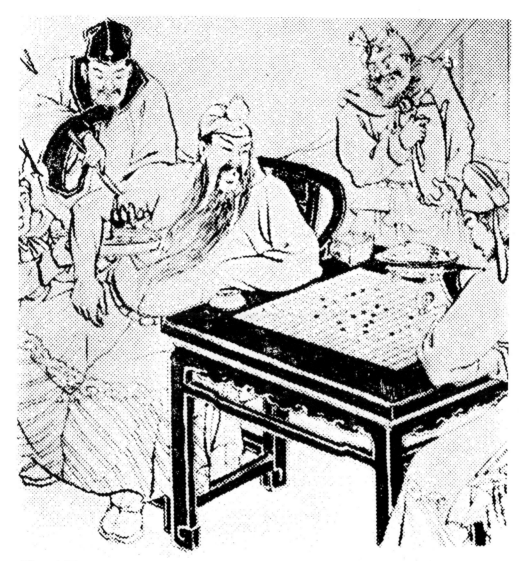

Plate 6. Hwa To, the first Chinese surgeon, removing an arrow from the arm of General Kuan Yu. (From Chen: *History of Chinese medical science*, 1969).

few far-sighted men, such as Viceroy Mendoza and the Franciscan monk Bernardino de Sahagún, attempted to save and reconstruct the remaining fragments of culture, but only nineteen texts from the whole body of Aztec writings were saved, and only eight texts of the Mixtec people.

Nicholas Monardes, a physician of Seville, published in three parts in 1565 a book on the medical methods and remedies of the natives of Mexico. He carried out experiments with several hundred Aztec and Mexican drugs, applying them in the treatment of his patients as the Aztecs had done for centuries. His successes were noteworthy, causing a mild sensation. Philip II, perhaps with a foresight heightened by guilt, commissioned Francisco Hernández to compile a work on the natural history of the New World, which comprised twenty-four books, and ten volumes of pictures and described 120 drugs and other remedies used by the Aztecs. The work was actually published in 1628, but in a greatly abbreviated form, Philip II having been dead for thirty years.

In 1743 Pierre Barrère, a French physician, published *Nouvelle relation de la France equinoxiale*, in which were depicted illustrations of a rubber ball, a rubber ring, and a rubber enema syringe, all of which he had found in South America, and were made and used by the Indians. Fifty years were to elapse before rubber surgical and medical appliances appeared in the catalogue of the London instrument makers, Savinier.

A purely Mexican herbal of the sixteenth century was discovered in the Vatican Library by Charles Upson Clark. This is known as the Badianus Manuscript, and represents the only medical text known to be the work of the Aztec Indians. It was written in Aztec by Martín de la Cruz, and was translated into Latin by Juannes Badianus, another Indian. The manuscript is on European-made paper, and was beautifully reproduced in colour facsimile in 1940, with a translation in English by Emily Walcott Emmart. Another translation, by William Gates, was published in 1939 by the Maya Society as *The De la Cruz-Badiano Aztec herbal of 1552*.

Both the Aztec and Mayan cultures had their origins in the Olmec civilization of the southern coastal region of the Gulf of Mexico. The Spaniards had begun their conquest of the Yucatán peninsula in 1524, and by 1546 Francisco de Montejo finally succeeded in subjugating the Mayan peoples of Yucatán. Only three Mayan books escaped destruction by the Spaniards: these contained astronomical and religious material, but no medical or related work. The Mayan civilization can be dated accurately from hieroglyphs found on buildings and steles to as early as 3113 B.C., and the great cities and states of the Mayas flourished from at least 500 B.C. to 909 A.D.

In Peru, the Conquistadores found no writing in the Inca Empire. The quipu was the only type of record that existed among the Incas. Quipus were strings which were knotted at various intervals, and served only to record numbers and instructions, never attaining the status of a genuine script.

Greece is regarded as the most important contributor to the growth of knowledge in the medical sciences, although much of Ancient Greek medical lore is intrinsically bound up with mythology, and it is often difficult to separate the two. Apollo, physician to the gods, is also seen as the bringer of disease and death, whilst Artemis, his sister, is simultaneously protector of women and children, and the goddess of death. Asklepios (Aesculapius), the serpent-bearer (the symbol of eternal life), was raised to godhead through the fame of his healing powers. His wife Epione, soother of pain, and his sons, Machaon and Podalirius, were the healers of the Greek warriors in the Trojan War, Machaon being a surgeon, and Podalirius a physician. His daughters were Hygieia, the giver of good health, and Panacea, the curer of all ills.

Much of what we know about Greek medicine can be culled from the writings of the poet Homer (8th century B.C.), especially in terms of the medicine practised on the soldiers in the Trojan War, where the removal of arrows and spears, the arresting of haemorrhage, and the use of pain-killing drugs were vital to the maintenance of a fighting force. Homer mentions Egypt in the *Odyssey*, recording the many medicinal plants and herbs grown there. He also states that, "In Egypt, men are more skilled in medicine than any of the human kind."

32

Asklepios, later worshipped as the god of healing, was said to have founded the guild of physicians who called themselves Asclepiads. The most famous of this body was Hippocrates, who was born on the island of Cos about 460 B.C. and died in Larissa, Thessaly, about 375 B.C. It has been suggested (Pollak and Underwood, 1968), that Hippocrates was probably of the twentieth generation from Asklepios, and he is generally accredited with the formulation of the 'Oath of the Asclepiads', which formed part of a larger medical work known as the Hippocratic Corpus. This collection of fifty-two medical works on seventy-two scrolls formed part of the Pharaonic library of the third century B.C., and was housed in Alexandria. The first complete edition of this work was printed in Rome in 1525 as *Opera omnia*, a folio edited and translated by Fabius Calvus. An edition of the Greek text was published by Aldus in Venice, 1526.

Another important figure in Greek medicine and science was Aristotle of Stagira (384-322 B.C.), a pupil of Plato. He executed what were probably the first anatomical illustrations, based on his dissections of animals. The best editions of the collected works of Aristotle are the *Opera*, five volumes, Berlin, 1851-1870, with text in both Greek and Latin; and the *Works*, edited by J. A. Smith and W. D. Ross, in twelve volumes, Oxford, 1908-1952.

With the gradual decline of Greek society, the centre of learning, including medicine, moved to Alexandria about 300 B.C. Men such as the Greek physicians Herophilus of Chalcedon and Erasistratus of Chios (c. 310-250 B.C.) were able to practise the systematic dissection of the human body, which religious and popular odium and prejudice had forbidden, not only in Greece, but in all other parts of the world. Herophilus wrote treatises on anatomy, dietetics and midwifery, along with commentaries on some of the writings of Hippocrates. Erasistratus compiled two works on anatomy, two on hygiene, one on the cause of disease, and also works on fever, gout, dropsy and abdominal complaints. Even under the Roman Empire, the centre of medical learning at Alexandria maintained its importance, although with the subjugation of Greece into the Empire the new focus was shifted to Rome.

According to legend, the foundations of the Roman Empire were laid in 753 B.C., when Rome was founded. In the third century B.C., Greek medical art found its way into the Roman Empire, brought by the Greek physicians and household slaves, whose successes surpassed those of the existing practices of exorcism and folk-medicine. Before the Greek infiltration, the only serious attempts at healing by practical application were made by the Etruscans, a conquered people whose knowledge of herbal remedies was renowned. Despite this apparent lack of medical interest, the sophistication of Roman public hygiene surpassed that of other co-existing cultures to a vast degree, with its system of sewage drainage canals, the supervision of the sales of consumables, and the inauguration of public baths.

Initially, Greek "slave doctors" were privileged and respected members of Roman society, and much sought after by wealthy families. Gradually, however, under the scathing criticism of such powerful persuaders as Cato the Censor (234-149 B.C.) the Greek influence became synonymous with degradation and the growth of immorality, and it was not until 91 B.C. that the practice of the art of Greek medicine to the exclusion of all others came to stay. In that year, a Greek physician named Asclepiades, a man of great learning, established a medical practice in Rome, and began training students. He is believed to have written about twenty books, of which only fragments remain. With the success of Asclepiades came an influx of Egyptian and Jewish physicians, who trained or half-trained so many aspirants to the profession that Rome soon possessed the highest patient/doctor ratio in the ancient world, specialization being the accepted practice. Physicians once again became highly regarded, and in 46 B.C. Julius Caesar, in an attempt to curb the strain on the depleted public granaries, banished eighty thousand non-Roman citizens to the colonies, but allowed all physicians and teachers to remain.

The Greek physician Galen (129-199 A.D.) was surgeon to the gladiators in Pergamon, his birthplace, before he went to Rome. Eventually, outstanding medical practitioners could be rewarded either by the position of "archiator palatinus" (court physician), or "archiator popularis" (district physician).

Without doubt, Galen was the most important literary contributor to medicine from the Roman period, and his prolific and dogmatic writings remained standard works for centuries. He came to Rome in 162 A.D., and began writing his two major anatomical works, *On anatomical procedure*, and *On the uses of the parts of the body to man*, the latter work establishing him as the founder of experimental physiology. Altogether, his works comprise nine books on anatomy, seventeen on physiology, six on pathology, fourteen on therapeutics, and thirty on pharmacy. Several collections of his works, and translations of individual books have been published, and they influenced medical thought and writings for several hundred years.

Another important writer working in Rome was Soranus of Ephesus (98-138 A.D.), an authority on paediatrics, obstetrics and gynaecology, his writings being the main source of Eucharius Rösslin's *Roszgarten* (1513), and its translation into English as *The byrth of mankynd* (1540), which first became associated with the name of Thomas Raynalde in the 1545 edition. Among the original works of Soranus are *On bandages*; *On fractures*; a *Life of Hippocrates*; and *Gynaecia*, which was translated in English in 1956. It is believed that there were illustrations in the original manuscript of *Gynaecia*, but these have not survived.

Aulus Cornelius Celsus (25 B.C. — 50 A.D.) was a Roman writer on medicine, although he was possibly not a physician. His *De medicina* is a compilation in Latin, largely based on the writings of Hippocrates.

Most of the writings of significant medical men were later printed in numerous editions and translations, but many had circulated in manuscript form for many years. It is probable that few of the original manuscripts as written by their authors survived, and if these were illustrated by drawings or diagrams of any kind, these stood even less chance of survival at the hands of various copyists. Many Greek texts disappeared completely in the original language, but some survived by virtue of the fact that they had been translated into Arabic and, sometimes centuries later, were then translated into Latin. Arabian and Persian medicine was the main path along which the medical knowledge of late antiquity was conveyed into the late Middle Ages. It arose out of the translations of Greek medical literature, notably Galen, but was enhanced by the observations made by the Persian and Arab physicians themselves, until by about 1000 A.D. the age of Middle Eastern medicine had reached its zenith, and was unequalled anywhere in the world.

The occupation of Spain by the Moors, and the resultant Arab influence, provided Europe with the base on which to build its own medical foundations, and the physicians of the Western Caliphate were among the most noteworthy represented by Arab culture. One of these was a Jew, Moses Maimonides (Rabbi Moses ben Maimon, 1135-1204 A.D.), who was born at Cordova. His writings include ten medical treatises in Arabic, all probably written in Cairo, where Maimonides had become physician to the Sultan Saladin. His books were immediately translated into Hebrew, but printed editions were published in several other languages, including English. Albucasis (Abulkasim; Abul Qasim, 936-1013 A.D.) was born at Zahra, near Cordova, and was among the first medical authors to describe haemophilia, and the treatment of deformities of the mouth. He wrote *Al-Tasrif*, consisting of thirty treatises in three books based on Paul of Aegina. Sections of this have been translated and separately published since 1471.

The Arabs developed ophthalmic medicine and urinoscopy to a high degree, but saw their medical knowledge achieve immortality when, in the eleventh century, an Arab pharmacist, Constantine the African of Carthage (1015-1087 A.D.), arrived in Salerno, which already had a thriving medical school. He was converted to Christianity, entered the monastery of Monte Cassino, and spent the rest of his life translating into Latin the medical literature of the Greeks and Arabs. Salerno became the new seat of medical learning, bringing together the best of the old world and forging the new, as had the Alexandrian school several hundred years earlier.

CHAPTER 3

MEDIAEVAL MANUSCRIPTS

"Probably the finest examples of illumination are to be found in the fifteenth century in France, Italy, England, and the Netherlands, though some still prefer the costly magnificent and florid ornamentation of the first quarter of the sixteenth century. The art is, however, generally in decline after about A.D. 1480."

Falconer Madan (1893).

Although historians tend to divide their subject up into compartments, the size of which is governed by centuries, reigns, wars, or other significant events, one must not look upon the subject as a sequence of happenings which started and ended abruptly. History is a continuous process which began before man acquired the gifts of reasoning and recording, and is still in progress. The evolution of any specific subject depends upon its origin and subsequent development, influenced by its environment and by the impact of events taking place elsewhere. A man's life does not begin with his birth; that is merely his acquisition of a separate existence. His physical death does not preclude his influencing people and events after his demise. Writings and drawings are two means by which a legacy can be left to posterity, but the material on which they are executed largely determines their survival.

Historians have tended to divide the subject into three sections: Ancient (up to *c.* A.D. 500), Mediaeval (*c.* 500-*c.* 1500), and Modern (*c.* 1500 to date). Manuscripts have been flourishing throughout the entire period since the introduction of papyrus, parchment and paper, and are still being produced. Theses and other writings on specialised subjects which publishers condemn as not being "financially viable", are deposited in universities and other institutions throughout the world, often in typescript, but sometimes handwritten, and with illustrations. Probably the most important period from the illustrations viewpoint was that generally known as "mediaeval", which has been arbitrarily defined as between about 500 to 1500. It will be noted that this extends to the end of the "incunabula" period covering the first fifty years of printing in Europe, which in fact saw the production of a large number of illuminated manuscripts, particularly in France.

The study of manuscripts is a highly specialized subject requiring a knowledge of palaeography, various languages, and of abbreviations used in the text. This is essential if the text describes the illustrations, the subject of which is not always obviously apparent. Medical subjects may not be familiar to the artist, and many of the illuminations display much detail not closely associated with the main subject. Clothing, furnishings, backgrounds and foregrounds are often of interest, but one must appreciate the fact that the illustrations and the actual text are not necessarily contemporary. For example, Greek authors might well be illustrated in the fifteenth century by French artists, in settings appropriate to that period.

Reproductions of the illustrations in mediaeval manuscripts, particularly in black-and-white, are very poor substitutes for those in the actual manuscripts. By their very nature, however, these exist in only one copy, and they are mainly scattered throughout the learned institutions of the world. This makes it very difficult to study particular items, but there is a large amount of literature devoted to the subject. Photographs of some of the miniatures have appeared in these, and in more general works on the history of medicine. The best book on medical illustrations in mediaeval manuscripts is that by Loren MacKinney (1965), who had spent thirty years studying medical manuscripts in Europe and the United States. All the important collections in the major centres of learning were explored, and the checklist of medical miniatures in extant manuscripts is particularly valuable. Entries are listed alphabetically by names of towns, and then by institutions, and all entries are dated, often approximately by century. The book is illustrated with 104 reproductions of miniatures, eighteen of which are in colour, and the select bibliography contains references to all the important books and articles written on the subject, indicating those which are particularly useful for their reproductions of miniatures. The illustrations are described in the text, which is divided into sections covering the following subjects: hospitals and clinics; diagnosis and prognosis by uroscopy, pulse-reading and astrology; materia medica; pharmacy; medication, external and internal; cauterization; bloodletting; surgery; orthopaedics; obstetrics; dentistry; bathing; veterinary medicine; and autopsy.

The Middle Ages was the most important period for beautifully-illustrated manuscripts, including many medical items in scripts not entirely devoted to medical subjects. Books on materia medica contain illustrations of animals and minerals, in addition to plants, and these "herbals" were popular and numerous. Illustrations were used from about 500 A.D. to illuminate texts, and a sixth-century Greek codex of Dioscorides' *Materia medica* with illustrations is preserved in Vienna. Ornamentation began with initial letters, the margins of the text, and then proceeded to miniatures. In Greece and Rome, scribes formed an important profession, and they survived for centuries in monasteries, where time was available to produce perfection in all forms of art and craft. Oak boards covered with leather, sometimes ornamented with precious stones and metals, were employed to bind the manuscripts, which were produced with lavish care. Red, blue and gold were primarily used for the illuminations, for which spaces were left by the scribe. Green, purple, yellow, white and black were also occasionally used for these unique decorations. The originals must be seen to be fully appreciated; coloured illustrations, if well produced photographically and by the latest colour printing techniques, must be the best substitute; and black-and-white reproductions can obviously give no idea of the richness of the colours, and the full beauty of the originals. Loren MacKinney (1965) provides illustrations of eighteen miniatures, and the same author (MacKinney, 1949) has contributed a synopsis of the history of ancient and mediaeval medical illustration. Falconer Madan (1893) wrote a useful introduction to the more general subject of books in manuscript.

Three illustrations from the fifteenth-century Mostyn MS.88 in the National Library of Wales have been reproduced by John Cule (1980), and show the table used in astrological medicine; the Zodiac Man, with Welsh instructions indicating times for avoiding venesection; and Welsh Bleeding Man, with instructions regarding diseases best treated by bleeding at particular sites.

When printing was first introduced, the earliest books closely resembled manuscripts, and sometimes included illustrations which had previously adorned the handwritten texts. An example of this is found in the compendium of anatomy of Mondino de' Luzzi, or Mundinus (c. 1275-1326), a native of Bologna. This was completed in 1316, and dominated the teaching of anatomy for over two hundred years. As *Anathomia*, it was first published in Pavia in 1478, and in Leipzig in 1493, subsequently going into numerous editions and translations, including one into English by Charles Singer in 1925. A rare edition by Johannes Adelphus was published as *De omnibus humani corporis interioribus menbris [sic. membris] Anathomia*, Strasbourg, 1513, a small quarto containing a small woodcut in the text, and a larger one on the last leaf. This represents a man with the thorax and abdomen dissected. The body is surrounded by ten medallions containing signs of the zodiac, two others of the signs being at the head and feet. Lines connect the organs of the body with the signs governing them (Plate 7).

A diagrammatic drawing of the female viscera with a fetus in the uterus (Plate 8) is featured in a miniature painted about 1400 A.D. (Leipzig MS. Codex 1122), being reproduced by Choulant (1945, facing p.84) from Karl Sudhoff's *Tradition und Naturbeobachtung*, Leipzig, 1907. This *Gravida* shows the traditional "frog-like" representation of the fetus as it was depicted for several hundred years, and not entirely replaced until the embryological drawings of Leonardo, Vesalius, Smellie and William Hunter became widely disseminated.

John Arderne (1307-c.1380) was one of the earliest recorded English surgeons, practising at Newark from 1349-1370 before coming to London. He had travelled widely as an army surgeon, and the results of his experiences were recorded in *A system of surgery* which consists of several separate treatises. At least sixty manuscripts of his writings exist, twenty-two being in the British Museum, others being at Oxford, Cambridge, Paris and Dublin. None of his works was published until 1588, when John Read issued an abridgement of Arderne's *Treatise of the fistula* in *A most excellent and compendious method of curing woundes in the head, and other partes of the body*, London, 1588. Arderne's work on fistula in ano, with its frequently reproduced illustrations, is his best known work, and translations of this and of *De arte physicali et de cirurgia*, have been published by Sir D'Arcy Power. A section on medical ethics has been translated by Paul Swain (1966), who also reproduced four illustrations from Arderne's writings. Two of these are particularly interesting because they show the body of a man bisected longitudinally, one from the front and the other through the spine (Plate 9). Dated 1412, these are very early examples of dissection scenes.

Mundini

Diſtincrio Neruorum

Neruí a cerebro. vij.paria Nuche colli vij.

Nuche ſpondiliũ pectorƺ.rij Nuche alchatyn v

Nuche alhouyns iij Nuche alhoſos iij

Et vnum impar.

Summa omnium neruoƺ rrrviij. Et vnũ impar:

Impreſſit Argentine Martinus Flach
Anno domini. M.D.riij.

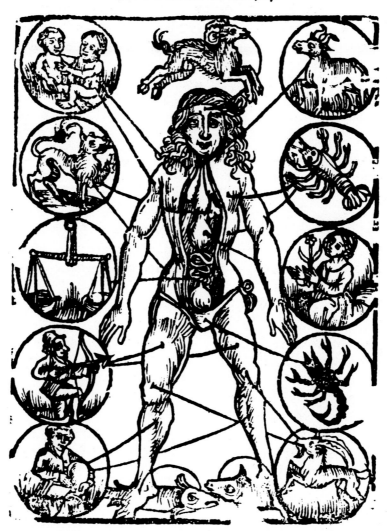

Plate 7. Illustration from *Anathomia*, 1513, by Mondino de' Luzzi
(*c*. 1275-1326), which had appeared in manuscripts of his work written
in 1316.

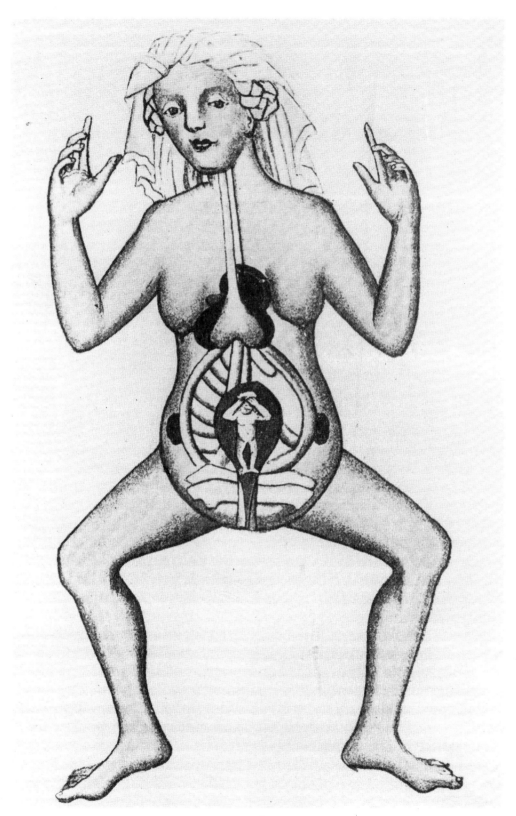

Plate 8. *Gravida.* From a miniature painted about 1400 A.D., in a Leipzig MS. Codex 1122.
(From Karl Sudhoff's *Tradition und Naturbeobachtung*, Leipzig, 1907; reproduced by Choulant,
1945, facing p. 84).

40

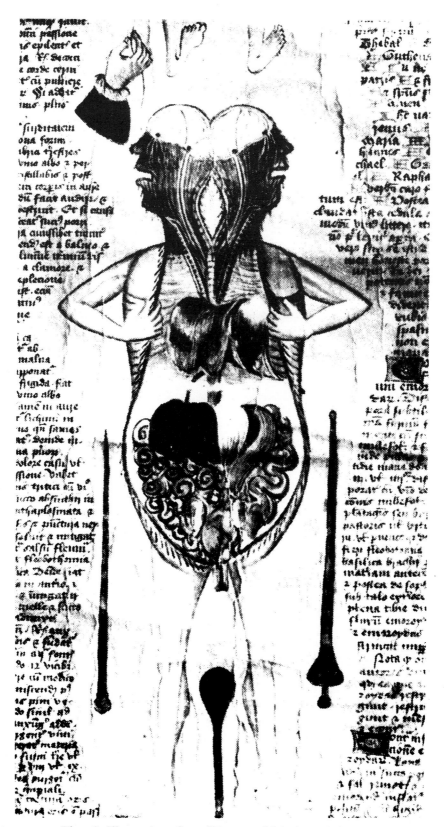

Plate 9. Illustrations from "De arte phisicale et de cirurgia,"
by John Arderne, dated 1412. (Wellcome Institute for the
History of Medicine).

Catalogues of manuscripts contained in the larger libraries are useful guides to the location of medical manuscripts containing illustrations. The British Library is an obvious repository for manuscript material, and contains many medical items; the Wellcome Institute for the History of Medicine has also published catalogues of manuscripts preserved there. S. A. J. Moorat's *Catalogue of Western manuscripts on medicine and science in the Wellcome Historical Medical Library. ... I. MSS. written before 1650 A.D.*, London, 1962 is particularly useful. It contains 800 entries comprising about 1500 individual works, with a coloured frontispiece, but no other illustrations. However, among the numerous indexes provided is one of MSS. in order of date, and a list of MSS. containing illustrations. This was followed by a second part, *II. MSS. written after 1650 A.D.*, which is divided into two volumes (A-M and N-Z), both published in 1973. It is arranged on a similar plan, describing over 4,000 manuscripts. These catalogues include full details of the manuscripts, including information on drawings and other illustrations in the texts, and various useful indexes.

Several other libraries have published separate catalogues of manuscripts, while others have included this material in general catalogues, occasionally in a separate section from the printed material. Such lists are invaluable to those attempting to locate manuscript material, which is elusive but often rewarding to those in search of illustrations in mediaeval manuscripts.

CHAPTER 4

THE INVENTION OF PRINTING AND THE SIXTEENTH CENTURY

"Books of the early presses have a flavour all their own, less personal perhaps than that roused by manuscripts, but of even greater intensity as illustrating the origin and evolution of the art which, more than any other, has set free the human mind."

Sir William Osler.

Without doubt the invention of printing was the most significant technological advance in the history of civilization. The diffusion of knowledge by word of mouth, letter writing, and the laborious copying and circulation of manuscripts, was replaced by the comparatively rapid duplication of copies by printing presses, still manually operated of course, but producing texts by the page, instead of letter-by-letter. The invention of paper in China, probably in A.D. 105, was a significant contribution, and a block-printed book, the Diamond Sutra, was also produced in China, in A.D. 868. Pi Sheng (*c.* 1041-1048) is said to have invented movable type, and the earliest extant book printed in this manner is the Korean *Sonja sail kaju*, which is dated 1409. Books by T. F. Carter (1955) and by Tsuen-Hsuin Tsien (1962) provide scholarly surveys of the history of book production and printing in China, but the spread of the methods of technology were slow in reaching Europe through the Arabs. In fact, the invention of printing from movable type was discovered and developed independently by Johann Gutenberg in Mainz. The art was perfected in 1450 after several years of experiment, and spread to Strassburg (1458), Bamberg (1461) and Cologne (1465). By 1500 fifty-one German towns housed printing presses, by which time the technique had spread into Italy, with presses in Subiaco (1465), Rome (1467), Venice (1469), and in 1471 presses were established in Milan, Florence and Naples. In France, printing was introduced at the Sorbonne in 1470, Switzerland had a press at Basle in 1468, and in Spain there was a press in Valencia in 1474. William Caxton (*c.* 1422–*c.* 1491) learned the art of printing in Cologne, and established a press at Bruges, where the first book printed in English was published in 1474. Two years later Caxton returned to England and set up a press in Westminster. Harry G. Aldis (1941) has provided a brief survey of the development and spread of printing in his *The printed book*, and the history of printing is the subject of many other monographs, including E. Gordon Duff's *Early printed books* (1893), and Alfred W. Pollard's *Early illustrated books* (1893).

Books printed in the fifteenth century are generally known as "incunabula", and they resembled the manuscripts they were replacing, the type-faces closely

43

following calligraphy, with spaces left for the rubrication of initial letters and other ornamentation. The colophon printed at the end of the work contained information regarding the title, author, name of printer, his device, and the date, although some of these details were often omitted. Title-pages did not come into general use until about 1480. It has been estimated by Aldis that editions of 38,000 books were printed in the fifteenth century, indicating the popularity achieved by printed works, which filled the needs of students and scholars, particularly in the university towns, where many of the presses were established. International trade in printed literature soon flourished. About 1461 books began to be illustrated with woodcuts, which could be printed simultaneously with the text. Some of the earliest medical items to be printed were semi-popular works in the form of purgation calendars, or broadsides, many of which bore astronomical figures or zodiacal men, the first piece of medical printing being one of these, the *Mainz Kalendar*, issued in 1457. This gives approximate dates for bleeding and purging, but although forty-six of these calendars were published before 1480, and about a hundred before the end of the century, copies of them are very rare. "Pestblätter", or plague tracts, were also common in the fifteenth century, and several studies of these forerunners of medical books have been made (see Thornton, 1966, pp.29-30).

Drawings of plants are featured in early manuscripts, in paintings by great artists, and were represented in the early printed herbals, where the illustrations were primarily intended to enable readers to identify medicinal plants. They were extensively used in domestic medicine, and although many of the early illustrations were very crude, the subject developed into medical botany, pharmacology and therapeutics. Several books have been devoted to the study of herbals, which are more closely related to the history of botany than of medicine, and the literature of the subject can be traced in Wilfrid Blunt's (1950) *The art of botanical illustration*. That book should be studied by all interested in the illustration of scientific subjects, since it is a veritable mine of information on a subject common to most sciences.

Yet another form of medical literature was issued as pictorial representations of dissections, the "graphic incunabula" of anatomy. These plates were either used individually for teaching, or sold as sets between covers. The dual publication of atlases as either separate plates or as collections was mainly due to economic factors, but the "collections" were often broken up and the plates (often framed and glazed) were displayed for teaching purposes in dissection rooms. The *Fasciculus medicinae* of Johannes de Ketham (died *c.* 1490) is an early example of medical literature containing a collection of short treatises on various specialist subjects, and is the first medical book to be illustrated by woodcuts. First printed in Venice in 1491, it went into many editions and translations, and the illustrations are very primitive, since they were not based on actual dissections, but feature the signs of the zodiac, sites for venesection, and the various parts liable to injury by a variety of weapons, these being depicted. The first Latin edition of 1491 is larger in format than later printings, and the woodcuts are on a bigger scale. They are not cross-hatched, and were probably intended to be coloured by hand. A dissection scene is depicted in Plate 10.

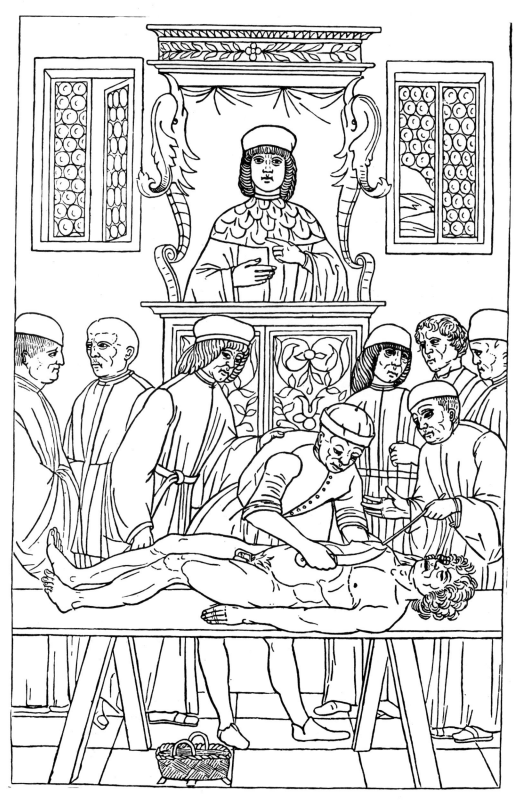

Plate 10. Illustration from Johannes de Ketham's *Fasciculus medicinae*, 1491, which contains the earliest anatomical woodcuts.

Leonardo da Vinci (1452-1519), a contemporary of Johannes de Ketham, is notable not only as a supreme artist, but as a scientist and anatomist. Unfortunately, his contributions to anatomy and other subjects were published posthumously.

However, the early painters greatly influenced those depicting medical subjects. These were often artists themselves engaged in copying paintings or engraving them for sale to art collectors. They copied the voluptuous figures of females and cherubs, posing these in statuesque postures amid unrealistic backgrounds, without apparently appreciating the incongruity of smiling creatures standing amid plants and animals while holding open their abdomens to display the anatomical details of their most intimate contents. This feature persisted in anatomical illustration for many years: Robert Knox (1791-1862) drew attention to this artistic licence in his *Great artists and great anatomists* (1852). Knox had seen the drawings of Leonardo at Windsor Castle, and in his book took the opportunity of giving advice which could be taken by all depicting anatomical structures. Knox (1852) wrote:

> "A knowledge of the interior of man's structure is essential to the surgeon and physician, to the zoologist and to the transcendental anatomist; it furnishes to the artist, as its highest aim, a *theory of art*. Hitherto, though not in all instances, it has unhappily induced the artist to display what he knows instead of enabling him cunningly to conceal that knowledge, as Nature has done, from the gaze of the world. He begins where he should end, and by drawing anatomically he displays that knowledge which he should keep in reserve merely to prove the correctness of his power of observing living forms." (pp. 144–5).

> "On the other hand, certain artists, following Angelo, endeavour to give a life-like appearance to their figures by putting in action all the superficial muscles. The result is, an *anatomical study* — a *galvanised corpse*. Follow Da Vinci. Draw the dead as dead — the living as living; never depart from the truth. The dissected muscle, besides being dead, is quite unlike the living in form, and in every other quality." (pp. 165-6).

Knox had very different views on Michelangelo (Michelagniolo Buonarroti Simoni) (1474-1564):

> "In the life and labours of Michael Angelo, we have an instance of the misapplication of Science to Art. He studied anatomy, and for a long time misunderstood its true relation to Art. This grand error he partly corrected towards the close of life, but it is doubtful if he ever wholly overcame it. Nor can I discover that deep, exact, and truthful character which characterized all Leonardo's labours". (p. 185).

Raphael Santi (Raffaello Sanzio) (1483-1520) was praised by Knox for the factual representation of his subjects:

"His knowledge of form, of proportions, and his perception of truth were absolutely perfect". (p. 188).

"Of anatomy he knew nothing, and must have been quite sensible of the misdirection of Angelo's studies. Whilst with other artists a life-like appearance is held to be of importance, with Raphael it was everything". (p. 189).

"His knowledge of the nude figure was not derived from anatomy, but from the study of living forms". (p. 195).

Knox had a final word of advice which should be considered by all medical artists:

"Learn anatomy by all means, but do not forget its object. When you draw a dissected limb be sure to sketch the living one beside it, that you may at once contrast them and note the differences". (pp. 202-3).

Thomas E. Keys (1940) has published a survey of medical books published in the fifteenth century, and a study by J. L. Thornton (1966, Chapter 2, pp. 27-39) provides additional information on sources of further information on the subject, including bibliographies, catalogues, and on the locations of collections of this material. In his *Incunabula scientifica et medica*, Bruges, 1938, Arnold Klebs listed over 850 editions of medical books printed before 1501, and 632 items are listed in F. N. L. Poynter's *A catalogue of incunabula in the Wellcome Historical Medical Library*, London, 1954. The latter is only one example of catalogues of collections of incunabula held in the larger medical libraries, but it is significant both for the extent of the collection and for the information provided with each entry, particularly regarding illustrations and ornamentation. Although printed illustrations in fifteenth-century books were confined to woodcuts, a few items were later rubricated, and initial capitals as well as the woodcuts were coloured. Capitals, for example, were sometimes coloured alternately in red and blue. Plate 11 is an example of a woodcut illustrating the title-page of a plague tract by Philippus Culmacher (*fl.* 1495) entitled *Regimen wider die Pestilenz*, [Leipzig, *c.* 1495]. This depicts St. Roch, and the figure of Death with a scythe, seated among the dead and dying. Plate 12 is a more delicately-executed woodcut on the title-page of Petrus Hispanus, Pope John XXI (died 1277): *Thesaurus pauperum*, [Florence, *c.* 1485], translated into Italian by Zucchero Bencivenni. This shows two surgeons operating on the head and leg respectively of two seated, fully-dressed patients.

Medical incunabula were often confined to printed versions of the classics which had hitherto circulated in manuscript form, and contain little original material. The woodcuts, for example, were usually copies of those to be found in manuscripts. Not being based on original research, they did not contribute to our knowledge of internal anatomy, for example, and although some are excellent examples of the art of the woodcutter, they were included more to attract the eye of the customer than to illustrate the text.

The illustrations in sixteenth-century books initiated the development of

Regimen zu deutsch Magistri philippi Culmachers võ Eger

wider die graufamen erfchrecklichenn Zötlichen peftelentz. von vil groffen meiftern gefamelt auß= getzogen: do durch fich ein menfch tzu peftelentz tzeit: nicht allein enthalden. Sunder auch wol gefreyen kan: gegeßen allen menfchen zu fundern nutz vnd groffer woltat.

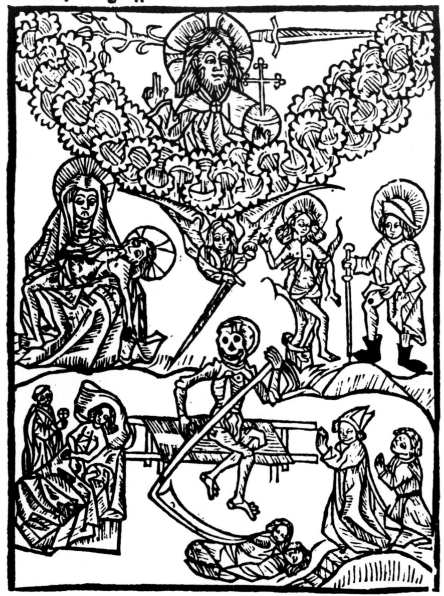

Plate 11. Woodcut of plague tract from Philippus Culmacher's *Regimen wider die Pestilenz*, [Leipzig, *c.* 1495]. (Wellcome Institute for the History of Medicine.)

48

truly scientific drawings which were essential to the text, and in fact the texts have sometimes survived mainly because of the plates. It is unfortunate that the anatomical drawings of Leonardo da Vinci (1452-1519) were not published during his lifetime, for they were more accurate anatomically than anything previously published. He wrote notes on painting, later published as the *Trattato della pittura* (1651), and mentioned the preparation of a textbook on human anatomy, but this was not published, and his drawings were not made generally available during his lifetime. Although these cannot be considered as examples of early medical book illustration, the history of their preparation and subsequent dispersal is fascinating. A collection of them was discovered many years afterwards in the Royal Collection. William Hunter (1718-1783) saw them there, and intended to publish them. Robert Knox, who saw them later, was equally impressed by their scientific value as supreme examples of anatomical investigation before the advent of Andreas Vesalius (1514-1564). There have since been published several collections of Leonardo's drawings, most of which are rare and expensive, but the first attempt at a systematic arrangement of the plates, with a new translation of the text was made by Charles D. O'Malley and J. B. de C. M. Saunders (1952). A useful study of Leonardo's life and work was published by Ludwig Goldscheider (1959), who includes a chronology of his life, and a short bibliography. Lindsey Pegus (1978) has contributed an article on the anatomical drawings.

During his lifetime Leonardo dissected thirty human corpses and many animals, his anatomical work probably extending from 1472 to 1519. He emphasized the value of pictorial description over the written word, and his drawings reveal not only structure but function. He illustrated most of the bones in the body, their action, the double curvature of the spine, the tilt of the pelvis, and the teeth. He sawed bones both longitudinally and in cross-section. Leonardo suggested a system of nomenclature for the muscles, of which he made a special study, and he recognized the heart as a muscle, being the first to describe it as four-chambered. These are but a few examples of his anatomical studies, which included the anatomy of the bat, horse, frog, bear, dog, and the wings of birds. Unfortunately, his studies of comparative anatomy led to some confusion in his drawings, and Elmer Belt, who amassed an enormous collection of Leonardo material, has suggested that in his magnificent drawing of the fetus *in utero*, the uterus is that of a cow (Belt, 1955, p. 19). Choulant, however, stated:

> "In scientific accuracy, these drawings eclipse those in Vesalius and are not approached in artistic beauty by anything before the time of Soemmerring and Scarpa. . . . He was the founder of physiological anatomy." (Choulant, 1945, p. 105).

Leonardo worked with a variety of materials, including silver-point on cream-coloured, red, or brownish paper, pen and ink, black or red chalk, and sometimes the drawings were heightened with white or with a wash.

The sixteenth century is of outstanding interest in the history of medicine on account of the anatomical studies of Vesalius, but before these were published

¶ Qui in comincia illibro chiamato theforo de poueri compilato et facto per maeftro pietro fpano.

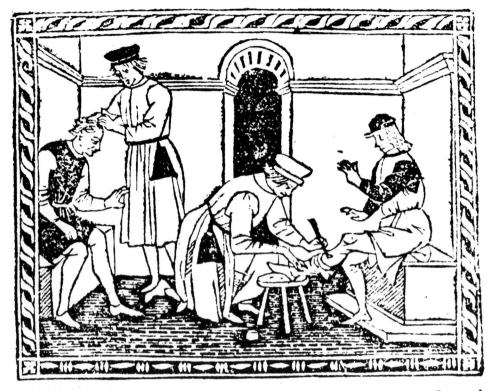

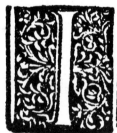 N nomine fancte & indiuidue trinitatis laquale creo tutte le cofe: & ciafcuna cofa doto di propria uirtute: & dallaquale ogni fapientia cidata a faui & lafcientia a faputi: opera comincio fopra le forze mie cofidandomi deilaiuto di celui fi come per noi p iftrumento adopera lopere fue tutte: laqle

Plate 12. Woodcut of operations, from Petrus Hispanus, Pope John XXI: *Thesaurus pauperum*, [Florence, *c.* 1485]. (Wellcome Institute for the History of Medicine).

there were a few notable items which are of interest for their impact from the medical illustration viewpoint. The earliest printed textbook for midwives was first published at Strassburg in 1513 as *De swangern frawen und hebammen Roszgarten*, and was written by Eucharius Rösslin (died 1526), a physician in Worms and later of Frankfurt-on-Main. This went into at least forty editions, and was translated into several languages. The book is illustrated with quaint fetal figures based on those in early manuscripts, which were probably derived from Soranus of Ephesus (A.D. 98-138), who practised in Rome. Rösslin's book was the first to be entirely devoted to obstetrics, and Plate 13 reproduces a woodcut of a bedchamber scene, and is taken from the Augsburg edition of

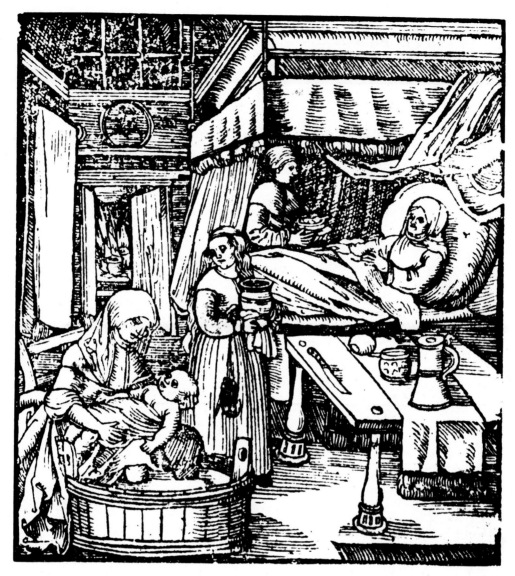

Plate 13. Woodcut of birth scene from Eucharius Rösslin's *Der schwangerenn frawen und hebammen Rosengarten*, Augsburg, 1541.

1541. An English translation, first published in 1540 as *The byrth of mankynd newly translated out of laten into Englysshe*, was the first work on midwifery to be published in English. This was issued in 1545 in an enlarged version, with an extensive prologue by Thomas Raynalde, "phisition", whose name appears on the title-page. The printer had the same name and was possibly related. These English editions contain copper-plate engravings of the woodcuts originally used in the *Roszgarten*, but with the addition of two anatomical figures based on those in the *Compendiosa totius anatomie delineatio, aere exarata*, 1545, by Thomas Geminus (died 1562), which derived from *De fabrica*, 1543, by Vesalius (see below).

It is of interest to note that the copper-engravings in *The byrth of mankynd* published up to 1545 were among the first in England to be produced by a roller press; also to note that later editions reverted to the use of woodcuts. With slight

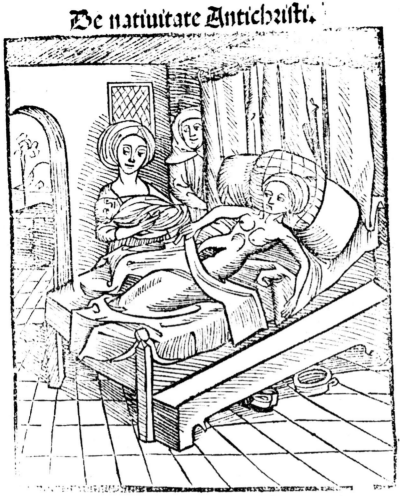

Plate 14. Woodcut showing the birth of Antichrist by Caesarean section, from Saint Methodius: *De revelatione facta ab angelo beato Methodio in carcere dento*, Basle, 1516.

variations in the title, and in the guise of translations and numerous editions, Rösslin's work, itself based on older material, persisted to influence midwifery for another century, and the illustrations adorned textbooks long after their authenticity had been disproved by the dissections of later anatomists. Jacob

Rueff (1500-1588), a Swiss obstetrician, published slightly amended versions of the fetal figures in his very popular textbook for midwives, *De conceptu et generatione hominis*, Frankfurt, 1580, but also added some original woodcuts. At least one of these was carved by Jost Amman (1539-1591), who included in the background an astrologer casting the horoscope of the baby. Both the Latin version of this, and a German translation, had first been published in 1554.

An illustration of particular obstetrical interest was contained in a non-medical book, and represents the birth of Antichrist by Caesarean section. It appears in Saint Methodius' *De revelatione facta ab angelo beato Methodio in carcere dento*, Basle, 1516 (d ii recto), the first edition of which was probably issued the previous year. This woodcut (Plate 14) was a very early representation of Caesarean section.

Although Hieronymus Brunschwig's *Buch der Cirurgia*, Strassburg, 1497, in its translation as *The noble handwork of surgery*, Southwark, 1525, was the first printed English surgery book, it did not contain the same woodcut illustrations as the German edition. The English publisher used more practical woodcuts which had been published in Hans von Gersdorff's *Feldbuch der Wundartzney*, Strassburg, 1517, but the English blocks are poor copies of the originals, some of which were attributed to Hans von Wächtlin of Basle. Gersdorff's book was printed by Johannes Schott, who was also responsible for the second edition published in 1526. Both editions contain twenty-five woodcuts illustrating military surgery, including amputation and surgical instruments, mostly full-page, with other decorative woodcuts. In the 1526 edition, the woodcut battlefield scene on the title-page is printed in red and black, the imposition of the red ink being crude. The illustrations in the 1517 edition have line borders around the blocks, which are otherwise identical with those in the 1526 edition. These are probably the best surgical illustrations of the period, and are notable also for the detail incorporated by the woodcutter in many of the scenes (Plate 15).

Albrecht Dürer (1471-1528) wrote many treatises on scientific subjects, but only two of his 150 books were printed during his lifetime. Famed as an artist, he was one of the first to practise the rules of perspective, and his book on human proportions was a great influence on all who recognised the fact that many drawings and paintings of human figures were unnatural, and sometimes grotesquely inaccurate. The depiction of medical subjects as illustrations in books necessitated complete accuracy, and this was facilitated by the publication of Dürer's work on the principles of proportion as applied to the human body. This was published shortly after his death, by his widow, and was prepared for the press by his friend Willibald Pirckheimer, to whom the book was dedicated. It bears the title *Hierin sind begriffen vier Bücher von menschlicher Proportion durch Albrechten Dürer zu Nuremberg erfunden und beschriben zu Nutz allen denen, so zu dieser Kunst lieb tragen*, Nuremberg, 1528, and it went into numerous editions and translations during both the sixteenth and seventeeth centuries. An illustration from the 1528 edition (Plate 16) shows a diagrammatic representation of a male; this book greatly influenced later artists representing human figures of both sexes, and of differing somatotypes.

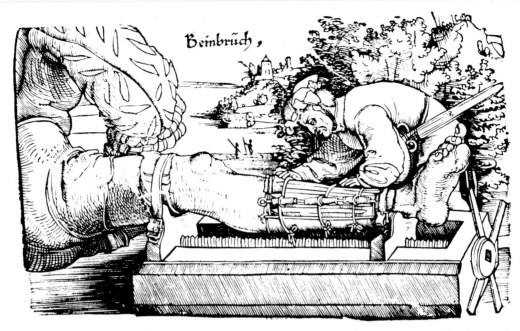

Beinbruch,

Plate 15. Woodcut of military surgery, from Hans von Gersdorff: *Feldbuch der Wundartznei*,
Strasbourg, 1526.

Although not published until two years after Vesalius' *De fabrica*, a book by
Charles Estienne (Stephanus) (1504-1564) was in preparation several years
before it was printed. This was *De dissectione partium corporis humani*, Paris,
1545, a French version of which was published in the following year. Printed by
Simon de Colines, the step-father of Charles Estienne, himself at one time
foreman in his brother's printing firm, and descended from a famous printing
family, this costly production was a fine example of the printer's craft. Estienne
had been assisted in his dissections by Etienne Rivière, a surgeon, who also
drew some of the illustrations. Many of the plates are dated between 1530 and
1532, and the work was completed up to the middle of the third book as early as
1539. A dispute between Estienne and Rivière delayed publication until two
years after *De fabrica*, (1543), but it can justly be described as pre-Vesalian. The
illustrations in *De dissectione* are the same in the Latin and French versions
except for the first five plates. The French version has sixty-three, one more
than the Latin text, and there are many other illustrations in the text.
Apparently the text is more instructive than the illustrations and was probably
revised after these were drawn. Many of them were the work of François Jollat,
a wood engraver whose work was well known in Paris between 1502 and 1550.
Some of the illustrations also appear to have been updated, but by means of
inset woodcuts, which are inferior to the original plates.

The figures are sometimes grotesquely posed in peculiar settings, and there
are many non-essential details included. For example, the entire figure of a
male nude is seated on a bolster at a window. The top half of his head is lacking,
exposing the cross-section of the brain, for which legends are provided in a
separate key. This very small section is the sole purpose for the large, elaborate
illustration (Plate 17).

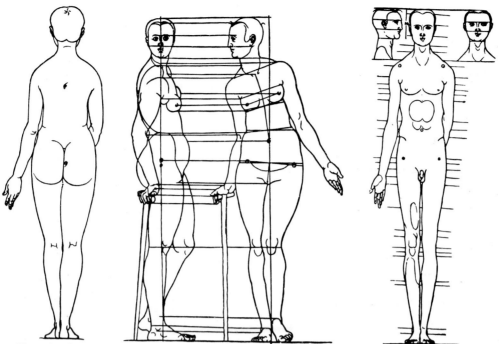

Plate 16. Woodcut by Albrecht Dürer, from his *Hierin sind begriffen vier Bücher von menschlicher Proportion*, Nuremberg, 1528.

Andreas Vesalius (1514-1564) was the first eminent anatomist to apply scientific methods to the study of his subject, and to publish his findings for the benefit of others. His anatomical writings with their outstanding illustrations form a landmark in the history of anatomy, and *De fabrica* was the outstanding medical publication of the sixteenth century. Vesalius was born in Brussels and, after studying medicine at Louvain and Paris, where he was a pupil of Jacobus Sylvius (1478-1555), he taught anatomy at Louvain before becoming professor of anatomy at Padua in 1537. He also taught anatomy simultaneously at Bologna and Pisa, but his association with Padua resulted in that school of medicine's gaining a world-wide reputation. Vesalius surreptitiously dissected the corpses of many executed criminals, among other subjects, gaining experience which made him increasingly dissatisfied with the teachings of Galen that then held sway in all spheres of medical education. Vesalius decided to write a textbook on anatomy incorporating the result of his researches, and spent many years on the project. He was the author of several other publications before *De fabrica* finally appeared in 1543, including *Tabulae anatomicae sex*, Venice, 1538, a very rare item, of which several facsimiles have been published, though as the title states, it contains only six plates.

The main work of Vesalius, *De humani corporis fabrica libri septem*, Basle, 1543, is usually known as *De fabrica*. This contains 663 folio pages, and over 300 illustrations, the best known being the page-size skeletons and "muscle-men". The decorated woodcut initials are also an outstanding feature, and have been the subject of studies by Robert Ollerenshaw (1952), and by Samuel W. Lambert *et al.* (1952, pp. 1-24). Lambert was also responsible for tracing some of the original blocks for the illustrations in *De fabrica* in Munich (Lambert *et al.* 1952, pp. 25-42), and all the original blocks were used for the publication of

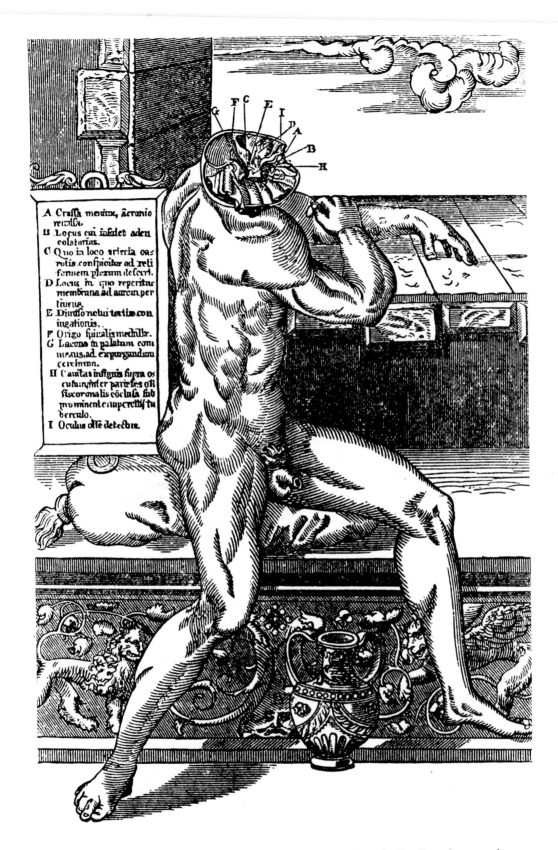

Plate 17. Wood-engraving from Charles Estienne [Stephanus]: *De dissectione partium corporis humani*, Paris, 1545.

Icones anatomicae of Andreas Vesalius, 1934 [1935], which was sponsored by the New York Academy of Medicine. The blocks were finally destroyed in Munich during World War II. The blocks for the initial letters did not survive with those for the main illustrations, and were probably part of the printer's stock, though they do not appear to have been used in any other book. Ollerenshaw (1952) has reproduced all the initial letters from the 1555 edition of *De fabrica*, which are superior to those in the 1543 edition. It is unlikely that the originals were drawn by Calcar, but they were probably executed for Oporinus in Basle, to match the type size, there being three main sets. As a background to each letter, cherubs (*putti*) are represented performing various anatomical and surgical operations.

During the same month of publication as *De fabrica* appeared the *Epitome* with the title *Suorum de humani corporis fabrica librorum epitome*, Basle, 1543. The male and female nudes, often referred to as "Adam and Eve", appeared only in the *Epitome*, and were in a chapter giving a brief enumeration of the terms used to describe surface anatomy (Frontispiece). Variations of these figures were reproduced in many other works; sometimes the male has an apple in his hand instead of a skull. The *Epitome* was intended more as an introduction to *De fabrica* for students than as a digest but, being much cheaper, it was more popular than the larger work. There have been many editions, translations and facsimiles of these and other books by Vesalius, and the plates were copied by many later anatomists. Some were flagrant plagiarisms of the originals, others were based upon them, and most give no recognition to their original sources. Their influence on medical illustration for several centuries was profound, and their importance in the history of anatomy cannot be over-emphasized. Sir William Osler once described *De fabrica* as "the greatest medical work ever printed", while K. Bryn Thomas (1974) has suggested that "the great anatomical folios began with Vesalius in 1543 and ended with William Hunter in 1774."

Although these books are known by the names of their authors, we must remember that at their instigation many others were involved in the production of the books as published. The dissections were drawn by artists, the drawings were carved or engraved, the text and blocks were reproduced by printers having great experience of their craft. The combined experience of the finest craftsmen resulted in books which have survived as magnificent specimens of book-production of the period, and there is honour sufficient for all participants to share. Unfortunately, very few of the older medical books contain any reference to the artists responsible for their illustrations, so that one must look to other sources for confirmation, or even hints, that particular artists made the drawings or engraved the blocks. This has resulted in a great deal of speculation and little positive proof, and even where much has been written about a particular author, as with Vesalius, it is extremely difficult to arrive at positive conclusions based on such conflicting views.

Vesalius was himself a capable artist, carefully supervising every stage in the production of his publications. At one time it was suggested that Titian was responsible for the drawings in *De fabrica* but it is most probable that one of his pupils, Jan Steven van Calcar (1499-1546) made at least three of the six drawings in the *Tabulae sex* published in 1538, and most of those for *De humani corporis fabrica*, first printed in 1543. The blocks were also cut in Venice, and were of pear wood sawed with the grain, and then treated with hot linseed oil. The woodcutting was performed by Francesco Marcolini da Forlì (*c.* 1505-*c.* 1560), an outstanding craftsman of the period. In a well-documented study, Francisco Guerra (1969) has made a scholarly investigation into the identity of the artists involved in *De fabrica*, 1543, correcting errors perpetrated by earlier writers on the subject. Charles D. O'Malley (1964) has provided much information in his extensive study of the life of Vesalius, which is also well documented and illustrated, and J. B. de C. M. Saunders and C. D. O'Malley (1973) have also reproduced the illustrations from the works of Vesalius. The study was first published in 1950, and contains annotations, translations, and a discussion of the plates and their background, with a biographical sketch of Vesalius. Another particularly important publication from the bio-bibliographical viewpoint was that by Harvey Cushing (1962), containing a facsimile of the 1543 edition of *De fabrica*, a list of Vesaliana published later, and many illustrations.

The text of *De fabrica* was completed in 1542, and Vesalius had obtained the services of the best artists and woodcutter to provide the illustrations. These were completed in Venice, but although there existed several fine printers in that city, Vesalius chose to print his masterpiece Joannes Oporinus (Herbst) (1507-1568) of Basle, a professor of Greek and Latin, and a keen scholar with some medical knowledge, who had become involved in a partnership of printers. After Oporinus became sole proprietor, his press gained an international reputation for the quality of its work. He was eminently qualified to undertake the gigantic task of publishing *De fabrica*, and was bold enough to take the risk. Vesalius first sent the text, followed by the woodcuts with proofs of the blocks, and later went to Basle to see the book through the press, making amendments to both text and illustrations during the process. It was during this period that Vesalius dissected the body of a criminal and prepared the skeleton which is still preserved in the University of Basle. The first edition of *De fabrica*, was, according to the colophon, completed in June 1543, but bound copies do not appear to have been available for another two months. The second edition was published in 1555, and was re-set, with numerous additional illustrations and alterations to existing plates. The text was also revised, for although Vesalius remained a Galenist as a result of his early training, he did not hesitate to incorporate the knowledge gained as the result of his own investigations and reasoning. In successive editions of his books he updated both text and illustrations, and it was only his comparatively early death which prevented him from making additional discoveries. For a complete understanding of his contributions to scientific anatomy it is essential to consider the text of *De fabrica* together with the illustrations, since he was still updating the former after the blocks had been cut. This proves his work to be a complete, illustrated textbook, in contrast to several atlases published later which consist mainly of illustrations with brief explanations, although some of these had separately

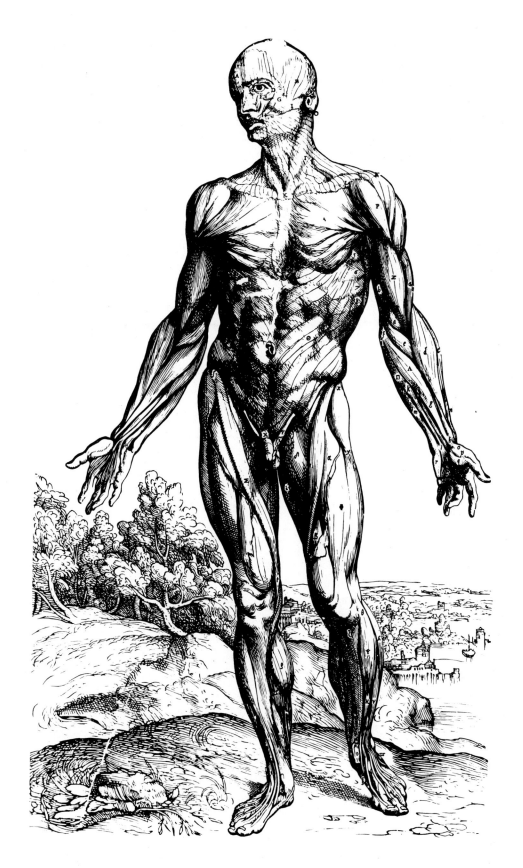

Plate 18. A "muscle man" from Andreas Vesalius: *De fabrica*, 1543.

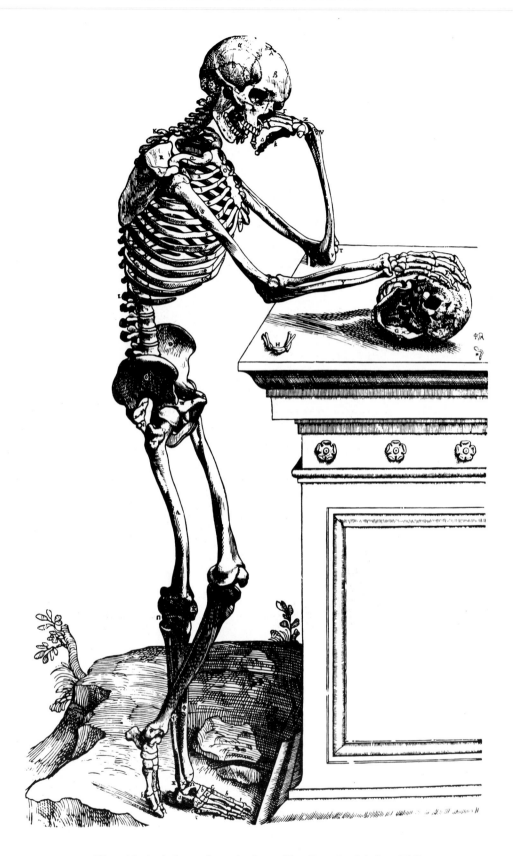

Plate 19. A skeleton from Andreas Vesalius: *De fabrica*, 1543.

published texts. These latter were often printed in a different format, and were often divorced from the atlases. Vesalius did not always appreciate the fact that, when the blocks were printed, the image would appear in reverse, and in the text there is sometimes confusion between left and right. When studying the large illustrations the foreground views will also be noted, and it has been discovered that when placed in correct sequence these form a continuous panorama, and the actual site has been identified. It is believed that these backgrounds were drawn by another artist, possibly Domenico Campagnola.

In the 1555 edition of *De fabrica* there is evidence of great improvement in the text and illustrations, and the book is much more attractive bibliographically. It is not so expensive on the rare book market as the 1543 edition, since collectors tend to place special value on first editions. However, it incorporates the corrections and additions made by the author, and the book is a credit to all concerned in its production. Plate 18 shows a full-length male figure displaying the superficial muscles, and Plate 19 represents a full-length skeleton viewed from the side, legs crossed, and standing beside a tomb. The head rests on the left hand, the elbow being on the tomb. The right hand rests on another skull on the tomb, on which are also drawings of the hyoid bone, and two ossicles of the middle ear, the malleus and the incus.

It is impossible to attempt to record the innumerable Vesalian copyists who closely followed his plates in their publications, sometimes in association with their own inferior illustrations. Some acknowledged their indebtedness to Vesalius, others neglected this courtesy, but they rapidly spread the new knowledge of scientific anatomy throughout the medical centres of Europe. Before the second edition of *De fabrica* was published, the plates of the 1543 edition were being copied in London, and were published in 1545. This was the first illustrated textbook of anatomy to be published in England, and the copper-plates with which it was illustrated were the first to be engraved there. The *Compendiosa totius anatomie delineatio* of Thomas Geminus (died 1562), London, 1545, was printed by Nicholas Hyll and published by John Herford. Geminus, a "foreigner" living in Leeds, was originally known as Thomas Lambrit (Lamberd; Lambert), and at one time set up as a surgeon. He was also an engraver, and executed the copper engravings, including the title-pages, with which the *Compendiosa* is illustrated. Henry VIII, to whom the book is dedicated, encouraged Geminus to publish the volume, which was translated into English by Nicholas Udall (died 1556), and published in 1553, the first edition being dedicated to Edward VI, and the third of 1559 to Elizabeth I. The first edition was printed by Geminus, who had set up a press in Blackfriars, and the same plates were used in all three editions, and in later French and German versions. The copperplates are not as clear and precise as the woodcuts in the original by Vesalius, and did not wear as well for successive impressions. LeRoy Crummer (1926) has suggested that Geminus engraved two of the plates in the second edition of Thomas Raynalde's *Byrth of mankynde*, published in 1545, using duplicate plates for his own book.

The writings of Walther Hermann Ryff are rare, and his reputation in the history of medicine has been tarnished by his plagiarism of the *Tabulae sex* of

Vesalius, and of *De historia stirpium*, Basle, 1542 by Leonhardt Fuchs (1501-1566). Ryff was the author of several other important books, one of the rarest being the first edition of his book on surgery, *Die gross Chirurgei oder volkomme Wundertznei*, Frankfurt, 1545. This contains numerous woodcuts depicting surgical operations and instruments, and the title-page includes a scene showing the amputation of a leg (Plate 20).

Another anatomist who was also a competent artist, made useful contributions to scientific anatomy, although he defended Galenic anatomy.

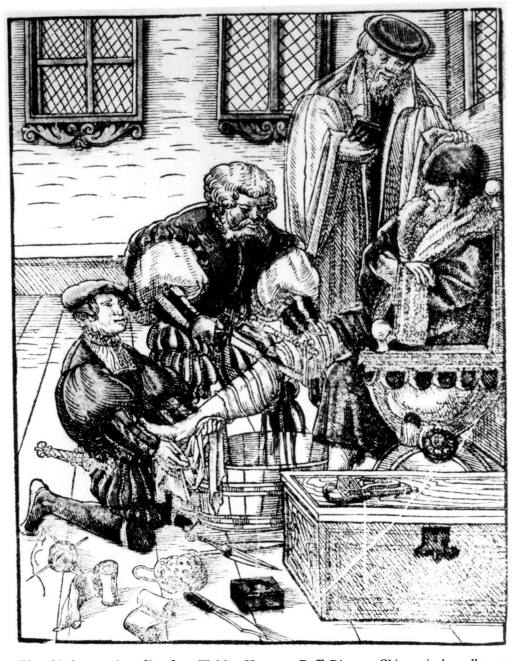

Plate 20. Amputation of leg, from Walther Hermann Ryff: *Die gross Chirurgei oder volkomme Wundertznei*, Frankfurt, 1545.

62

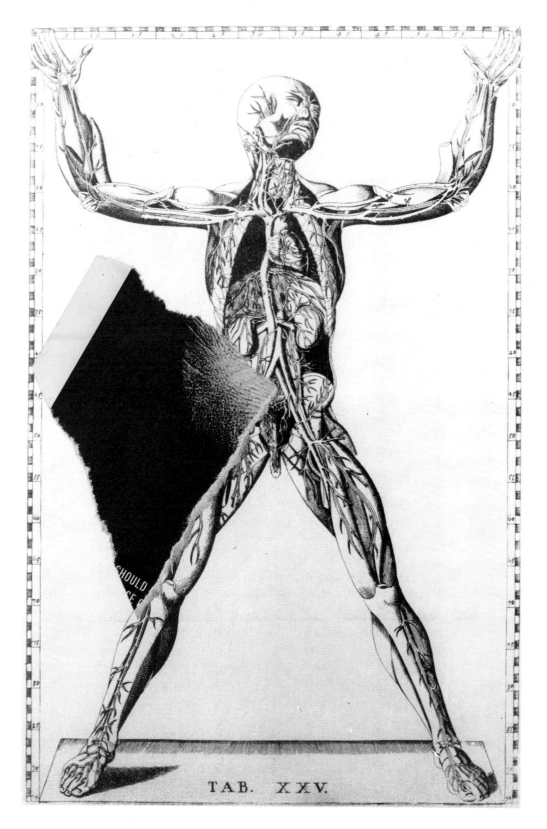

Plate 21. Copper-engraving probably made about 1552, with tables of measurements as borders, from Bartholommeo Eustachio: *Tabulae anatomicae*, Rome, 1714

Bartholommeo Eustachio (1520-1574) of Sanseverino made many of the drawings for his *Opuscula anatomica*, Venice, 1564, with a second edition, Leyden, 1707, and a third, Delft, 1726. Eustachio and his friend Pier Matteo Pini also made drawings for another book, but he died leaving the thirty-eight copperplates, which had been completed in 1552, to Pini. The plates later came into the hands of Giovanni Maria Lancisi, and they were published with eight others which had been printed in *Opuscula anatomica*, as *Tabulae anatomicae Bartholomaei Eustachii* [*etc.*], Rome, 1714. The illustrations, engraved on copper by Giulio de' Musi of Rome, are outstanding for their accuracy and precision. Eustachio disliked the method of printing letters on the figures featured in his illustrations so, as Plate 21 indicates, he used graduated margins. The parts and their names were found by means of a ruler, and some editions actually contained a ruler. This is similar to the use of map references, and can also function as a scale for measuring proportions. This book is another example of how posthumous publication of a work prevented due recognition's being accorded to the author during his liftime.

CHAPTER 5

THE SEVENTEENTH CENTURY

"The best work of the 17th century, whether of Shakespeare or Molière, Rembrandt or Velasquez, Spinoza or Newton, Harvey or Leeuwenhoek, was either conceived from some deep source of original inspiration or else sprang from a fresh, naive wonderment over the newly revealed marvels of nature, as when old Pepys declared himself 'with child' to see any new or strange thing".

Fielding Hudson Garrison.

Stimulated by the scientific methods of Vesalius and other anatomists of the previous century, medical men and scientists in general embarked on research in increasing numbers as the seventeenth century progressed. The writings of the pioneers quickly became available throughout the civilized world, either as original publications, or embellishing the writings of others. Both science and the arts advanced by rapid strides, although there remained an overlapping of traditional views with the new sciences, which had to be irrefutably substantiated before the older theories were finally abandoned. Alchemy gave way slowly to chemistry, but traces of magic and quackery persisted, and have never been completely eradicated, particularly where applied to therapeutics. The use of herbs with unknown properties and in haphazard mixtures continued to be popular until the standardization of drugs eventually brought some degree of control, but in the *London Pharmacopoeia* of 1618, worms and many other unsavoury ingredients were included. However, the foundation of new universities, the formation of scientific societies, and the advent of periodical literature, fostered the development of education, and stimulated research.

In the previous century, emphasis had been mainly on osteology, myology, the blood vessels and the gross anatomy of the main organs. A more scientific approach developed, and the interior of the body was more closely investigated (the brain, the heart, and the circulation of the blood) while the development of more powerful lenses led to microscopical examination of the tissues. The need for greater detail in illustrations was met by the emergence of the engraving as the successor to the woodcut in medical illustration, although the latter was to be employed again in the nineteenth century.

An early attempt at printing woodcuts in colour was made in Italy with the publication in 1627 of *De lactibus sive lacteis venis*, by Gasparo Aselli (1581-1626). This was printed in Milan, and contains the first description of the lacteal vessels. It contains four large foldout polychrome woodcuts in folio, black being used for the background, the contours, crosshatching, veins, and for the letters engraved on the figures; white, the colour of the paper, indicates the numbering of the plates on the black background, and for the chyliferous vessels; dark red was used for arteries, crosshatching and for shadows; and light red for the surface of the intestines, the mesentery and the liver. The organs represented are all animal, not human. The process of imposing the blocks in succession, allowing the sheets to dry between impressions, was both slow and expensive. It is significant that the plates were engraved and printed in black in later editions: multi-colour printing for medical illustrations was not attempted again for almost a century.

Another innovation which gained popularity in the seventeenth century was achieved by the superimposition of sections of plates. One of the most popular was *Catoptron microcosmicum* by Johann Remmelin (born 1583), first published, probably in Ulm, in 1613, but without his knowledge, and he published a corrected edition in 1619. The anatomical value of the work is very slight, and it was possibly intended for laymen rather than for medical students. Several editions and translations were published, the last as late as 1720. In the early editions the plates were engraved by Lucas Kilian (1579-1637) of Augsburg, and originally consisted of five copper-plates, which were cut up, and the smaller pictures superimposed on the male and female figures. The parts were then lying successively under each other, and could be lifted to reveal the various organs. The idea was later copied in a few other publications, and had been employed earlier in "fugitive sheets", but it mainly became popular in books for children.

Giulio Casserio of Piacenza, also known as Julius Casserius Placentinus (1561-1616), was a pupil of Hieronymus Fabricius ab Aquapendente, and succeeded him as professor of anatomy at Padua in 1604. He was the author of *De vocis audituseque organis historia anatomicae*, Ferrara, [1601], a large folio which contains thirty-seven copper-plates, for which both the drawings and engravings were executed by Joseph (Josias) Maurer. Twelve of the plates in this book appertaining to the ear, with twenty-one new ones depicting the other sense organs, were used in his *Pentaestheseion hoc est de quinque sensibus liber*, Venice, 1609, but a second edition, published in Frankfurt in 1622 with a different title, is in smaller format with reduced plates by another artist. About 1600, Casserius planned a larger work covering the entire field of human anatomy, but unfortunately he died before it was completed. Adriaan van der Spieghel, known as Spigelius (1578-1625), succeeded Casserius at Padua, and prepared several texts before his death, requesting Rindfleisch, generally known as Bucretius, to publish them. These works were not illustrated, but Bucretius asked the heirs of Casserius for the unpublished plates left by him, intending to use them to illustrate the manuscripts left by Spigelius. Casserius received seventy-eight plates, and used seventy-seven of them, together with twenty others, to publish them as *Julii Casserii Placentini Tabulae anatomicae LXXIIX, omnes novae nec antehac visae; Dan. Bucretius XX quae deerant supplevit et omnium explicationes addidit*, Venice, 1627, Odoardo Fialetti (1573-1638) and Francesco Valegio (Valesius) being named on the copper-engraved title as respective artist and engraver. These plates were also used in the first edition of the anatomy book planned by Spigelius, which was published as *De humani corporis fabrica libri decem*, Venice, 1627.

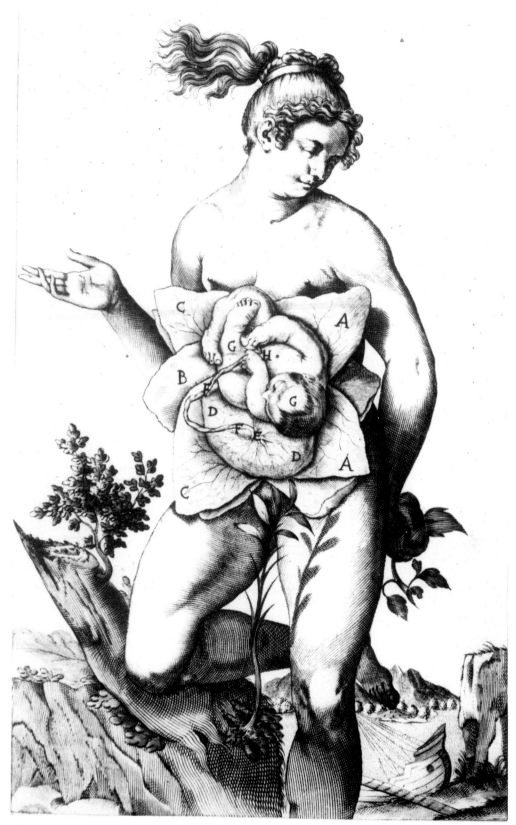

Plate 22. Female, with fetus still attached to the placenta, placed on abdomen. Prepared for
Julius Casserius, but eventually published in Spigelius: *De formatu foetu*, Padua, [1626].

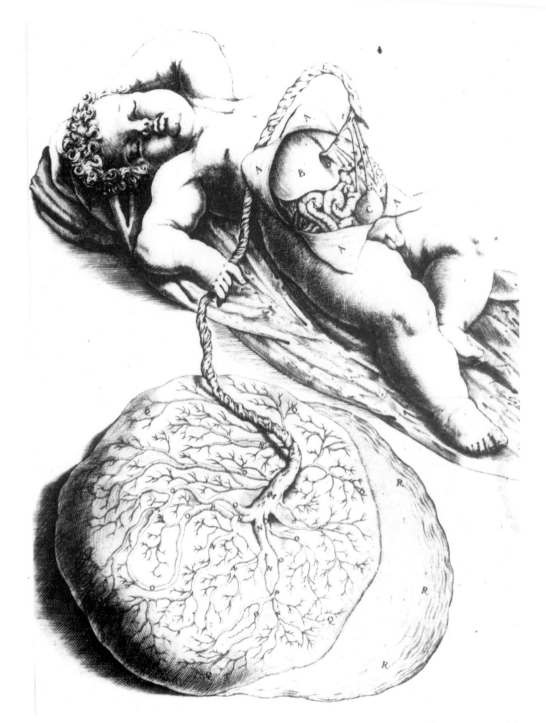

Plate 23. Fetus and placenta, showing connections from the placenta to the fetus. Prepared for Julius Casserius, but eventually published in Spigelius: *De formatu foetu*, Padua, [1626].

Liberalis Crema, a son-in-law of Spigelius, had bought other copper-plates from the grandson of Casserius, and when he published a selection from the posthumous works of Spigelius, Crema selected nine plates and published them in *Adriani Spigelii De formatu foetu*, [*etc.*], Padua, [1626]. The illustrations

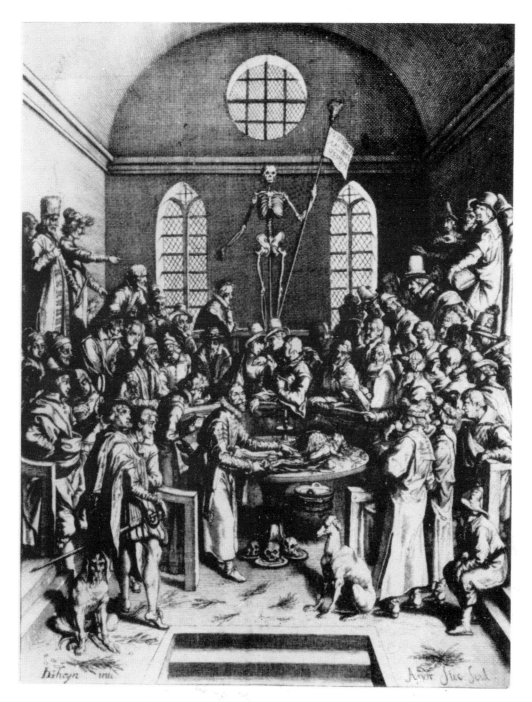

Plate 24. Anatomical theatre at Leyden, with dissection scene, from Pieter Pauw (or Paaw): *Succenturiatus anatomicus*, Leyden, 1616.

have been described as the most beautiful of the plates left by Casserius, and this edition is very rare (Plates 22-23). The complete works of Spigelius were published by Joannes Antonides van der Linden (1609-1664) as *Adriani Spigelii Opera quae extant omnia. Ex recensione Joh. Antonidae van der Linden*, two volumes, Amsterdam, 1645. These superbly-printed volumes contain the ninety-seven anatomical plates originally published, the twenty added by

69

Bucretius, the nine used in *De formatu foetu*, and another featuring the hymen, also from the Casserius collection. Other plates illustrating some of the writings of Gasparo Aselli, William Harvey, Johannes Wallaeus and others, which are also featured in the book, were included. This widespread use of the copper-plates engraved for Casserius, covering the whole field of human anatomy, ensured that they became models for future anatomists, not only for their technical accuracy, but for the artistic beauty of their reproduction as copper-plates. Despite the peak of success reached by the woodcuts in *De fabrica* by Vesalius, that method of reproduction was demonstrated as being surpassed by copper-engravings at their best.

Another pupil of Fabricius, Pieter Pauw or Paaw (1564–1617), became professor of anatomy at Leyden, where he built the anatomy theatre featured in the frontispiece of his book, *Succenturiatus anatomicus continens commentaria in Hippocratem, de capitis vulveribus additae in aliquot capita libri VIII. C. Celsi explicationes*, Leyden, 1616 (Plate 24). This shows Pauw dissecting, and is similar in design to the title-page of *De fabrica*. The book is devoted to the anatomy and surgery of the head, containing fine illustrations of the head, brain, teeth, and surgical instruments. Pauw also wrote the commentary to an edition of Vesalius' *Epitome*, published in 1616, in which the original illustrations were replaced by small engraved copper-plates.

Most of the books mentioned were large, imposing tomes, with plates outstanding for their artistic merit or their subject matter. However, probably the most significant book in the history of medicine was published in the seventeenth century in a rather mean format, replete with typographical errors, and illustrated with copper-plates copied from another source. This was the first and best-known book by William Harvey, published as *Exercitationes anatomica de motu cordis et sanguinis in animalibus*, Frankfurt, 1628. In this he first demonstrated the circulation of the blood, and the illustrations form an

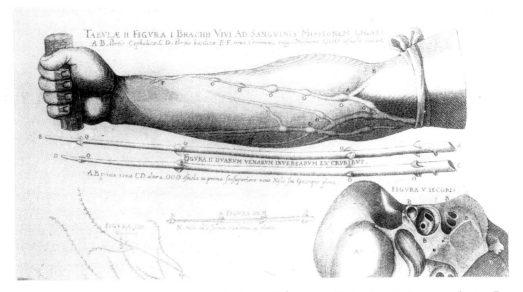

Plate 25. Valves in the veins of the arm, from Hieronymus Fabricius ab Aquapendente: *De venarum ostiolis*, Padua, 1603.

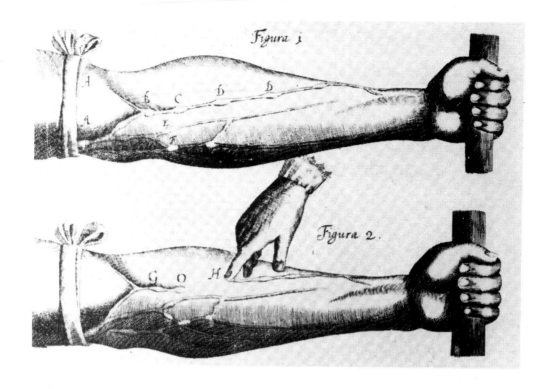

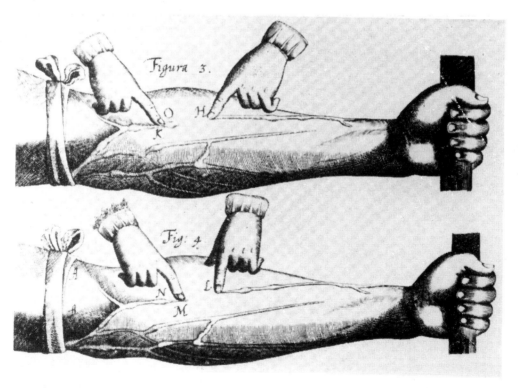

Plate 26. Valves in the veins of the arm, as copied from Fabricius in William Harvey: *De motu cordis*, Frankfurt, 1628.

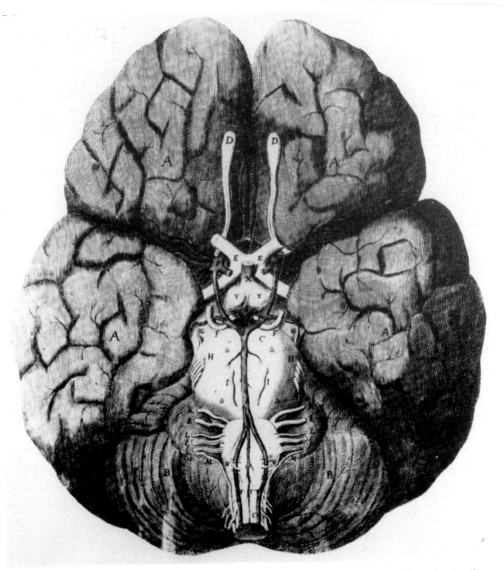

Plate 27. Engraving of drawing by [Sir] Christopher Wren of the base of the brain, from Thomas Willis: *Cerebri anatome*, London, 1664.

essential part of his thesis, clarifying, even for the lay person, a text which is in itself a careful exposition, but depends on the plates for confirmation at a glance. William Harvey (1578-1657) was born in Folkestone, and after his theoretical medical education at Cambridge, proceeded to Padua for the completion of his studies. At his arrival there early in 1600, Hieronymus Fabricius ab Aquapendente (Girolamo Fabrizio, 1536-1619) had been lecturing for many years. He claimed to have seen the valves in the veins as early as 1574, and had probably demonstrated them in his lectures. However, it was not until Harvey had left Padua that Fabricius published *De venarum ostiolis*, Padua, 1603, but he did not understand their true function, and he was not the first to see them. However, his tract of 1603 was illustrated with an engraving demonstrating the valves in the veins (Plate 25), which was later copied in *De motu cordis* by his former pupil William Harvey.

72

Harvey's *De motu cordis* of 1628 contained sixty-eight pages of type, meanly printed on poor paper (with the exception of a few copies), and with many typographical errors, some of which were corrected by means of an errata slip inserted in some of the copies. The two engraved plates, which were reproduced in all later editions except the first English translation published in 1653, were probably engraved in Frankfurt, where the book was published (Plate 26), but comparison with Plate 25 indicates their close resemblance. The reason why Harvey's book was published in Frankfurt is probably explained by the fact that Robert Fludd (1574-1637), a friend of Harvey, and the author of several books, had sent them for publication to Johann Theodore de Bry in Frankfurt. De Bry died in 1626, and William Fitzer, an Englishman who married de Bry's daughter in 1625, succeeded to the publishing business. Publishing on the Continent was more flourishing than in England, and apparently authors were better treated. Fludd (quoted by Keynes, 1966, p. 176) complained that:

> ". . . home-born Printers demanded of me five hundred pounds to print the first volume and to find the cuts in copper; but beyond the seas, it was printed at no cost of mine, and that as I could wish. And I had 16 copies sent me over, with 40 pounds in gold as my gratuity for it."

No doubt Fludd's experience persuaded Harvey to have his work published abroad, although unfortunately he was not able to see it through the press. If the printer had to set the book in type from Harvey's handwriting, which was execrable, the long list of errata is readily explained. However, this does not detract from the value of the book as a pioneer in the history of physiology, and a model of scientific investigation. Yet, while Harvey argued that the blood finds its way from the right ventricle through the parenchyma of the lungs into the pulmonary vein and left ventricle, he never saw the capillaries. He knew they must be there, but was unable to demonstrate them because he did not have a sufficiently powerful lens to identify them. A definitive life of William Harvey has been written by Sir Geoffrey Keynes (1966), who also compiled a comprehensive bibliography of Harvey's writings (Keynes, 1953), both of which provide further information on *De motu cordis*. Harvey's work on the circulation of the blood is also the subject of an interesting study by Gweneth Whitteridge (1971).

Thomas Willis (1621-1675) was the author of several books, but he is best known for his work on the nervous system. In 1660 he became Sedleian Professor of Natural Philosophy at Oxford, and during this period he was assisted in his experiments by Richard Lower, Thomas Millington, and Christopher Wren, who made drawings for Willis. As Sir Christopher Wren (1632-1723) he is mainly remembered as the architect responsible for the building of St. Paul's Cathedral, but he also made important contributions to astronomy, mathematics and other branches of science. He made drawings of minute bodies under the microscope, removed the spleens of dogs, injected liquids into the veins of dogs and performed other scientific experiments. His early career as a scientist has been recorded in a "popular" biography by Harold

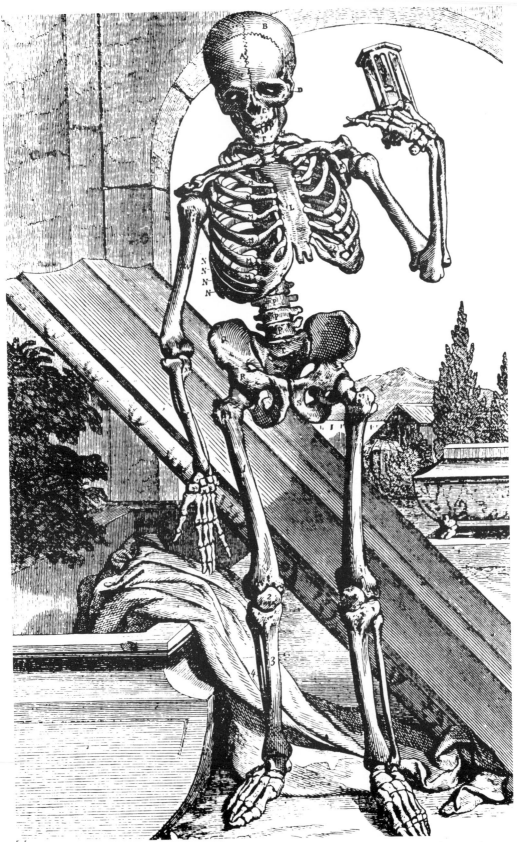

Plate 28. Copper-plate of skeleton from Godfried Bidloo: *Anatomia humani corporis*,
Amsterdam, 1685.

F. Hutchison (1975), and William C. Gibson (1970) has reproduced a watercolour, signed by Wren and Willis, which is in the Wellcome Institute for the History of Medicine. This depicts a section of the small intestine, and is but one of many drawings made by Wren for Willis. Some of these were included in *Cerebri anatome nervorumque descripti et usus*, London, 1664, which contains a most accurate description of the nervous system, and describes the "nerve of Willis", and the "circle of Willis" (Plate 27).

Godfried Bidloo (1649-1713), a native of Amsterdam, was professor of anatomy at The Hague, and later at Leyden. He was the author of a large folio devoted to the entire field of human anatomy, entitled *Anatomia humani corporis*, [*etc.*] Amsterdam, 1685, which contains 105 anatomical copper-plates (Plate 28). The drawings were made by Gerard de Lairesse (1640-1711), but although they are artistically attractive, anatomically they are inferior to many earlier atlases. The plates engraved by the brothers Peter and Philip Van Gunst are good examples of the craft of copper-engraving, but the book was not well received by other anatomists, and it was not a financial success. Three hundred impressions of the plates were given to William Cowper (1666-1709) by the publisher, and Cowper later published them under his own name as *The anatomy of humane bodies*, [*etc.*], Oxford, 1697. This contains 105 of the plates drawn by Lairesse, and nine new plates drawn by Henry Cook, and engraved by Michiel van der Gucht. Cowper was also the author of *Myotomia reformata: or a new administration of all the muscles of the human body*, London, 1694, and after Cowper's death Richard Mead (1673-1754) paid for a sumptuously-produced new edition in 1724. This is the book which should commemorate William Cowper, rather than his being remembered as a plagiarist of Bidloo's plates.

Sebastian Christian a Zeidlern was the author of *Somatotomia anthropologica. Seu corporis humani fabrica methodice divisa, et controversarum quaestionum discussi*, Prague, 1686, which was published after his death, and was edited by his son, Bernard Norbert Zeidlern. In the engraved title-page the author is depicted demonstrating in the dissecting room at Prague (Plate 29). The book is a small folio with twenty-eight full-page, original copper-plates, and although the text mainly refers to Greek authorities, there are also references to the work of Vesalius, Columbus, Caspar Bartholinus, and Jean Fernel.

Despite the original research promoted by William Harvey's work on the circulation, the development of the microscope, and the publication of several outstanding books in other branches of science, there were comparatively few books on medical subjects containing noteworthy illustrations. Many of the anatomical texts were illustrated with plates copied from earlier writings, and most of the shorter communications were in the form of papers submitted to the Royal Society, founded in 1662, and published in its *Philosophical Transactions*. Similar societies were established in Italy, Germany, France, and most published their proceedings, some also sponsoring monographs. Although this led to an increase in the output of scientific literature, and a speedier diffusion of knowledge throughout Europe, it did have certain disadvantages. Unless

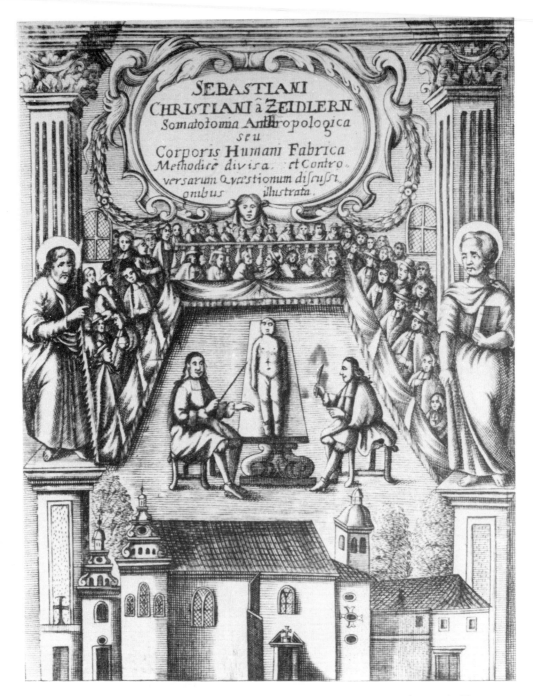

Plate 29. Sebastian Christian a Zeidlern demonstrating in a lecture theatre in Prague.
Engraved copper-plate of title from his *Somatotomia anthropologica*, Prague, 1686.

medical authors were wealthy enough to pay printers to publish their books, or
were prepared to send them abroad, where they might be welcomed,
particularly if the name of the author were well established, they stood little
chance of having their work printed. Many books remained in manuscript,
some were copied and circulated, and a few have survived in manuscript form in
the larger medical and university libraries.

76

CHAPTER 6

THE EIGHTEENTH CENTURY

"In this matter we have much to learn from the old printers, in whose books paper, type, illustrations, initial letters, and borders were all so planned as to form a harmonious whole".

Alfred W. Pollard (1893).

During the eighteenth century, medical books underwent a transformation which, although gradual at the beginning of the century, had significantly changed the techniques of book production by the end of that period. The decoration of books became more related to the proportions of the book both in size and typography. The crowded, heavily adorned title-pages, with engraved half-titles often including portraits of the authors, became displaced by simple vignettes, and the woodcut initial letters, head-pieces and tail-pieces gradually disappeared. However, woodcut decorations were very durable, and were often used in several publications. Seventeenth-century woodcuts can be found in eighteenth-century books. Ellen B. Wells (1970) has described these developments, and in a later article (Ellen B. Wells, 1976), has detailed the various techniques used in medical book illustration during the eighteenth century.

We have noted that probably the earliest attempts at colour printing were the woodcuts published in *De lactibus*, [*etc.*], Milan, 1627, by Gasparo Aselli (1581-1626). This pioneer effort was not pursued, and another venture into colour printing in medical books was also abortive. This was initiated in the early years of the eighteenth century by Jacques Christophe (or Jacob Christoph) Le Blon (or Le Blond) (1667-1741). Born at Frankfurt-on-Main, he is said to have studied engraving in Zürich under Conrad Meyer, and in Paris under Abraham Bosse, before he went in 1696 to Rome, where he studied painting under Carlo Maratti. There he met Bonaventura van Overbeek, the Dutch painter, and returned with him to Amsterdam, where Le Blon settled temporarily as a painter of miniature portraits. While in Amsterdam in 1704 he made his first attempts at producing coloured mezzotints, using blue, yellow and red. He later went to The Hague, Paris and London, where he attempted to patent his process. He established a wall-paper factory in London, but this failed and he returned to The Hague and then to Paris. There he eventually secured a patent for coloured copper printing, but died in 1741. Copies of prints executed by Le Blon are rare. Peter Krivatsy (1968) has provided information on Le Blon and the three anatomical plates known to have been executed by him. He had several pupils and assistants, and two of them continued in the attempt to apply coloured mezzotint engraving to the illustration of medical subjects.

Jan Ladmiral (1698-1773) was one of these, and he was born in Normandy. Both he and his brother Jacob were pupils of Le Blon when he was in London; Jan Ladmiral later claimed the invention of colour engraving as his own. He offered his service to Bernhard Siegfried Albinus, and six plates were published under the title *Anatomische voorwerpen door Jan Ladmiral* between 1736 and 1741, two with a text by Albinus, others showing preparations by Fredrik Ruysch (1638-1731), while the sixth appears to be an imitation of Le Blon's plate dated 1721, but with no mention of Le Blon.

Jacques Fabian Gautier d'Agoty (1710-1786) was born in Marseilles, where he met Le Blon, and later became his assistant. After the death of Le Blon, Gautier acquired his privilege in 1745, but he also claimed to be the inventor of coloured copper-plate printing. In fact, he only added a fourth black plate to the three colour plates used by Le Blon, and it is probable that even the latter himself employed the black plate. Gautier's plates are impressive in size, but the colours are sombre, and were not enhanced by the protective coats of varnish applied. He did most of the dissecting himself, and was also the artist and engraver. Some of his plates were used in successive publications, and *Myologie complètte en couleur et grandeur naturelle*, [etc.], Paris, 1746, (Plate 30) containing twenty plates, consists of two earlier publications, *Essai d'anatomie en tableaux imprimés, qui representent au naturel tous les muscles de la face, du col, de la tête, de la langue et du larinx, d'après les parties dessequées et preparées par L. Duverney, ... comprenant huit grandes planches dessinées, peintes, gravées et imprimées en couleur et grandeur naturelles par le Sieur Gautier*, [etc.] Paris, 1745, with eight plates; and *Suite de l'Essai d'anatomie*, [etc.] Paris, 1745, containing twelve plates. Gautier was also the author o *Anatomie de la tête*, [etc.], Paris, 1748, containing eight plates; *Anatomie générale des viscères*, Paris, 1752, with twenty-four plates; *Exposition anatomique de la structure du corps humain*, Marseilles, Paris and Amsterdam, 1759, with twenty plates; also of several other works on anatomy and natural history published between 1773 and 1775. In 1914, twelve unsigned painted panels attributed to Gautier d'Agoty were exhibited in Paris, and were possibly the originals of some of the plates in his publications. These panels are now in the Wellcome Institute for the History of Medicine. The plates are very rare, and were very costly to produce and publish. The time taken to engrave the three or four plates, each to be printed separately in turn, allowing the sheets to dry between the processes, followed by a coat of varnish, was considerable. Furthermore, the results would not have satisfied other authors or artists in search of techniques capable of expressing fine detail, for although colour can effectively be used for anatomical teaching purposes, there is little variation in the colours of post mortem tissues. It is significant that coloured engravings were not to become popular for medical illustrations, and that although mezzotint was successful for the reproduction of paintings and similar subjects, it does not appear to have been used for other medical subjects except by C. N. Jenty (see below). Pierre Pizon (1950) has published an interesting article on Gautier, giving details of his various publications, and reproducing seven of his illustrations.

The first half of the eighteenth century was singularly deficient in

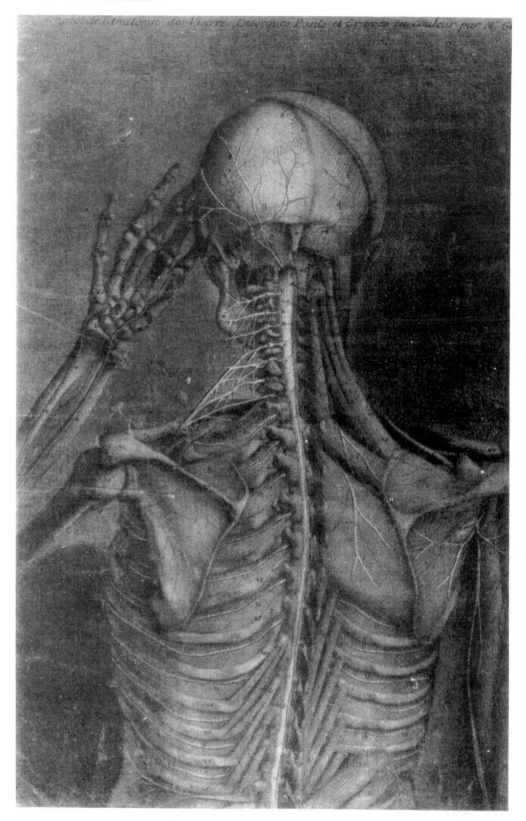

Plate 30. Illustration from the first anatomical atlas to be printed in colours. From Jacques Fabian Gautier-d'Agoty: *Myologie complète en couleur et grandeur naturelle*, Paris, 1746-1754.

outstanding medical publications. The great scientists and physicians of the previous century were either dead or in their final years, and although there were some outstanding physicians and surgeons on the Continent, those in England appeared to be exhausted by the frantic scientific activity of the period following the publication of William Harvey's *De motu cordis* in 1628, and the foundation of the Royal Society in 1662. A few outstanding physicians gained high reputations, and earned large sums of money, but those who wrote books added little to medical knowledge. William LeFanu (1972) in his Fielding H. Garrison Lecture for 1971 provides a masterly survey of this period, which he called "The lost half-century in English medicine". Books with outstanding illustrations were rare; on the English scene William Cheselden's books stand out above any other publications of the period.

William Cheselden (1688-1752) was a pupil of William Cowper at the age of fifteen, and eventually became surgeon to St. Thomas's Hospital. He was first noted as a lithotomist, publishing *A treatise on the high operation for the stone*, London, in 1723. He was already the author of *The anatomy of the humane body*, London, 1713, which became so popular as a textbook that it was published in numerous successive editions until the end of the century (Plate 31). His outstanding publication, *Osteographia*, which cost a vast sum of money to produce, achieved little success when issued in a strictly limited edition, but is now highly valued, mainly for its magnificent copper-plates. Cheselden planned his greatest work to appear in three volumes, but it was not completed. Subscriptions were invited at four guineas, and it was stipulated that only three hundred copies were to be printed in English, with a further one hundred sets of the plates for a Latin or French edition. The plates would then be destroyed. Only ninety-seven of the three hundred copies were sold, and Cheselden later broke up eighty-three copies to sell the plates separately, in an endeavour to recoup some of his expenditure. A unique copy of a trial issue is in the Hunterian Collection, Glasgow, and bears the title *The anatomy of the bones*, London, 1728, and lacks text or letter-press. Eventually the large folio was published as *Osteographia, or the anatomy of the bones*, London, 1733, and all complete copies contain two sets of plates, one lettered and the other unlettered. K. F. Russell (1954) has provided full bibliographical information on these issues.

The work contains fifty-six large plates, and forty-four smaller ornamental ones, the latter being mainly of skeletons of animals. Cheselden stated that most of the large plates were executed by Gerard Vandergucht (1696-1776), for whose work he had great admiration. In his Address to the Reader he wrote:

> "Two of the smaller plates, the head of the mantyger, and the sceleton of the tortoise, and all the large plates except xiii, xi, xxi, and xxxi were done by Mr. Gerard Vandergucht, and how great an artist he is, the open free stile in which these plates are etched and engraved, and the inimitable manner of expressing the different textures of the parts sufficiently show."

The rest of the illustrations were by "Mr. Shinevoet", identified by William

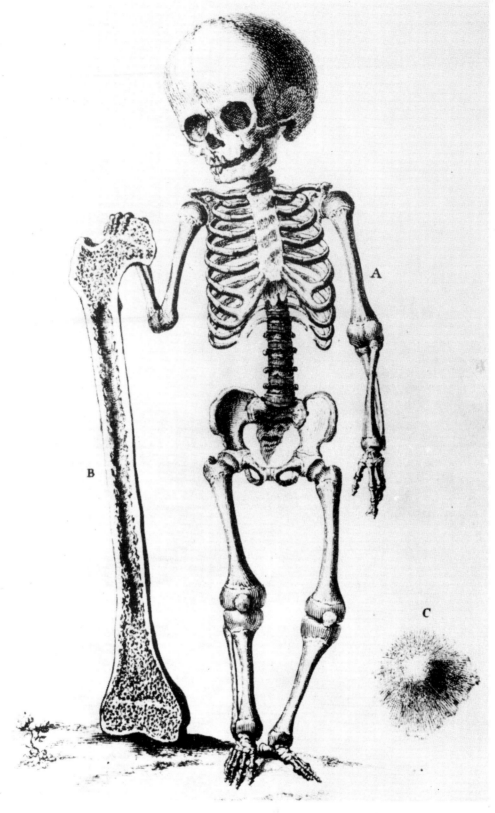

Plate 31. Skeleton of child, and internal structure of bone, drawn and engraved by Gerard van der Gucht. From William Cheselden: *The anatomy of the human body*, 5th ed., London, 1740.

LeFanu (1960) as Jacobus Schijnvoet (1685-1723), a native of Amsterdam then working in London on such subjects as drawings of the interiors of cathedrals. Before he had completed his work for Cheselden, Schijnvoet died, and in his Address to the Reader, Cheselden wrote of him:

> ". . . his manner of etching, though wonderfully neat and expressive, and so well suited to such things as he was mostly employed in, is nevertheless much inferior in stile to that of Mr. Vandergucht".

A vignette on the title-page of *Osteographia* shows the "camera obscura", as devised by Cheselden, possibly the first time it was employed for drawing medical subjects, although the principle had been in use for scientific purposes for several centuries. The vignette is said to show Cheselden with his face in the apparatus, drawing the subject, which is being arranged by his pupil, John Belchier. The latter wrote a review of the book (reproduced by K. F. Russell, 1954), which Belchier described as "being undoubtedly the most magnificent work of the kind now extant". The "camera obscura" enabled drawings to be executed more accurately and more expeditiously, and was an improvement on other methods of obtaining proportionate drawings. Robert Ollerenshaw (1977) has contributed an article on its earliest recorded use in medical illustration. Sir Zachary Cope (1953) was the author of a biography of William Cheselden, which contains full details of his life and publications. The original drawings by both Schijnvoet and Vandergucht were discovered in the Royal Academy, and were deposited in the Library of the Royal College of Surgeons of England.

Another anatomist, Bernhard Siegfried Albinus (1697-1770), was the author of several atlases which became famed for the beauty of the illustrations. A native of Frankfurt-on-the-Oder, he studied under Boerhaave in Leyden, moved to Paris, then returned to his native town to become professor of anatomy and surgery in 1721. He endeavoured to present scientific information in as much detail as possible, and set high standards for the accuracy of the illustrations to his books, reputedly spending 24,000 florins on these. Having secured the services of a skilled artist, Jan Wandelaer (1690-1759), Albinus scrupulously supervised his work. All the subjects were carefully measured and brought down to scale, and the illustrations were engraved directly on copper. Wandelaer had worked for Fredrik Ruysch and Arent Cant, and had been a pupil of Gerard de Lairesse, among others. He therefore had some anatomical knowledge, and used an ingenious device in the drawing of skeletons and muscles. Two large nets, divided into squares, were placed in front of the skeleton, one with a mesh one-tenth of the size of the other, about four feet from the other. The artist placed himself forty feet from the subject. Choulant (1945, p. 276) gives much information on the illustrations to the writings of Albinus, and also quotes the reply of Albinus to criticisms of Wandelaer's work by Pieter Camper.

Albinus was the author of numerous publications, the following being particularly noteworthy for their illustrations: *Historia musculorum hominis*,

Leyden, 1734, the eight plates in which were drawn and engraved by Wandelaer, although they do not bear his name; *Icones ossium foetus humani*, Leyden, 1737, with thirty-two copper-plates, only the first one bearing the name of Wandelaer, who engraved the plates directly from the preparations; *Tabulae sceleti et musculorum corporis humani*, Leyden, 1747, all the forty copper-plates of which bear the name of Wandelaer, in this principal work by Albinus (Plate 32); *Tabulae VII uteri mulieris gravidae cum jam parturiret mortuae*, Leyden, 1748, with seven copper-plates of the gravid uterus, and an *Appendix*, 1751, containing a single plate illustrating the fetus. *Tabulae ossium humanorum*, Leyden, 1753, which is a continuation of *Tabulae sceleti*, and contains seventy copper-plates; *Tabula vasis chyliferi cum vena Azyga, arteriis intercostalibus aliisque vicinis partibus*, Leyden, 1757, the single plate by Wandelaer consisting of a life-size representation of the thoracic duct; and *Academicarum annotationum libri I-VIII*, Leiden 1754-1768, in two volumes containing thirty-seven copper-plates, some of which bear Wandelaer's name. Choulant (1945, p. 283) mentioned when he was writing his original text that the original drawings executed by Jan Wandelaer for Albinus were in the Medico-Chirurgical Academy of Dresden.

Illustrations by Wandelaer were published in several other books, and there were many later imitations, mostly without acknowledgement, and inferior to the outstanding work of this brilliant artist. His engravings, which ensured the success of the atlases of Albinus, should certainly assure him of an eminent place among medical artists.

It will be appreciated that while some artists are noted for remarkable landscapes, portraits, still-lifes or other subjects, some are particularly appreciated for their treatment of hands, faces, drapes, or even backgrounds. Animal painters and botanical illustrators also tend to specialise in particular aspects of their chosen subjects, and it is impossible to select outstanding artists who are equally capable of depicting, with the same dexterity, every object capable of reproduction by crayon, pen or paintbrush. An example may be given of George Stubbs (1724-1806), famous as the author of *The anatomy of the horse*, 1766, and for his paintings of horses and other animals. He had an intimate knowledge of the anatomy of the horse, gained by careful dissection over many years. Stubbs had also studied human anatomy in York under Charles Atkinson, who also encouraged him to give lectures to medical students. John Burton (1710-1771) asked Stubbs to illustrate his book, *An essay towards a complete new system of midwifery*, London, 1751, so Stubbs taught himself the art of engraving for this purpose. The book contains eighteen engravings on copper, which are technically poor in quality, and are certainly not based on original observation. They do not bear Stubbs's name, and he could not have been proud of this venture into a subject with which he was unfamiliar. The engravings are reproduced in a book on Stubbs's anatomical works, by Terence Doherty (1974), and additional information on his life and paintings is available in a well-produced book by William Gaunt (1977). R. B. Fountain (1968), and William B. Ober (1970) have contributed shorter studies on his work.

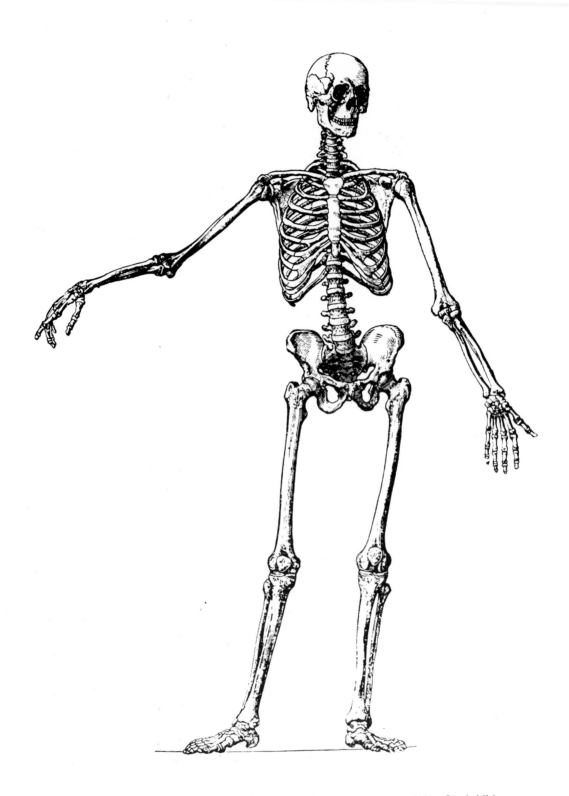

Plate 32. Engraving of skeleton by Jan Wandelaer, from Bernhard Siegfried Albinus:
Tabulae sceleti et musculorum corporis humani, Leyden, 1747.

The first half of the eighteenth century had produced very few well-illustrated medical books, but the next fifty years saw a great revival. In England one notes in particular the publication of the great obstetrical atlases of William Smellie, C. N. Jenty and William Hunter. These had in common the fact that Jan Van Rymsdyk (died 1788 or 1789) was the artist responsible for the drawings on which most of the illustrations to these atlases were based. The scanty known facts of his life, and information on his work, have been published in *Jan Van Rymsdyk, medical artist of the eighteenth century*, by John L. Thornton (1982), but a brief summary of his connection with the authors of these outstanding books is necessary to place in perspective his position among the outstanding medical artists of this period.

Jan Van Rymsdyk suddenly appeared in London in 1750, and although we know he had lived in Holland, we have little personal information on his career except such as can be gleaned from his *Museum Britannicum*, first published in 1778, and from his dated original drawings. We know nothing of his previous experience either as an artist or with the depiction of medical subjects, but he was obviously good enough at his work to satisfy the fastidious William Hunter, and the less demanding William Smellie. Rymsdyk was making drawings for William Hunter in 1750, William Smellie in 1751, and Charles Nicholas Jenty in 1757, all these being of the gravid uterus, and he returned to the same subject in 1784 when he made a similar drawing for Thomas Denman. These drawings have been compared in an article by J. L. Thornton and Patricia Want (1979), but for this particular purpose we shall deal with the illustrations chronologically according to the dates of publication of the books in which they were published.

William Smellie (1697-1763) practised in his native town Lanark from 1720 to 1739, when he went to London, and after a brief visit to Paris settled in London. Taking a modest house in Pall Mall, he set up as an apothecary and practitioner of midwifery, and began teaching midwifery in 1741. He took both male and female pupils, separately, taking his students to attend poor women in their own homes. Smellie contributed to the improvement of forceps, and formulated rules for their use. He was the author of the three-volume *Treatise on the theory and practice of midwifery*, published between 1752 and 1764, with varying titles for the second and third volumes. In the first one he had advertised an accompanying volume of plates in larger format, which was in active preparation. It was intended to contain twenty-six plates, according to the advertisement, but this was increased to thirty-nine, and Smellie stated in his Preface that he had originally planned to have "twenty-two, which Mr. Rymsdyke had finished above two years ago". This suggests that Rymsdyk had completed that number of drawings by 1752, as the atlas was published in 1754 as *A sett [sic] of anatomical tables with explanations and an abridgement of the practice of midwifery, with a view to illustrate a Treatise on the subject*, London. Rymsdyk made the drawings for twenty-five of the plates, all the originals being preserved in the Hunterian Collection, Glasgow. They were purchased by William Hunter at an auction in 1770 following the death of Dr. John Harvie, who had succeeded Smellie as teacher of midwifery in Wardour Street. Pieter

(Petrus) Camper (1722-1789), made drawings for Smellie in 1752 on one of his three visits to to England, eleven of these being engraved as illustrations for Smellie's atlas. The originals are now in the Library of the Royal College of Physicians of Edinburgh, most being signed by the artist and dated 1752. William Smellie mentions two plates as being by "another hand", but there were three (not two) not attributed to either Camper or Rymsdyk, and it is probable that Smellie himself drew them.

William Smellie stated in his Preface that the figures were mainly to explain his teaching to midwives, "avoiding however, the extreme Minutiae . . . the situation of parts and their respective dimensions being more particularly attended to than a minute anatomical investigation of their structure [etc.]". Rymsdyk's drawings were probably more explicit than Smellie required, and were certainly much more detailed than those executed by Camper. In fact, many by the latter are diagrammatic, and Grignion, the engraver, embellished the engravings with more detail than is included in Camper's original drawings.

Charles Grignion (or Grignon) (1717-1810) engraved all the plates in Smellie's *Atlas*, and also engraved a portrait of William Smellie, drawn or painted by Jan Van Rymsdyk in 1753. The location of the original is not known, and only two copies of the engraving have been traced. Charles Grignion was born in London, and studied under Hubert François Gravelot. At the age of sixteen he went to Paris to work under J. P. LeBas for six months, before returning to work under Gravelot and G. Scotin. In 1738 he set up as an engraver on his own account, illustrating many books, including one by Albinus published in 1757. He headed a school of engraving and enjoyed prosperity until his school was superseded, and he lived on charity in his old age. His nephew, Charles Grignion (1754-1804), received premiums at the Society of Arts in 1765 and 1768, during which period Andrew Van Rymsdyk (1753 or 4-1786), the son of Jan Van Rymsdyk, also received premiums there, and it is probable that the two families were closely acquainted.

Rymsdyk was also making drawings for John Hunter (1728-1793), many of which are preserved in the Library of the Royal College of Surgeons of England. Most were either not published, or were later used to illustrate papers published in periodicals. However, the first book published by John Hunter was *The natural history of the human teeth*, 1771, with a second part entitled *A practical treatise on the diseases of the teeth*, 1778. In his "advertisement" or preface, Hunter states that most of the observations in the book were made before 1755, when the figures were drawn by Rymsdyk. They were engraved by Strange, Grignion and others. The work contains sixteen plates, for which there are twenty-six original drawings, all housed at the Royal College of Surgeons. Additional information on Rymsdyk's work for John Hunter is available in J. L. Thornton's *Jan Van Rymsdyk* (1982).

Charles Nicholas Jenty, about whom little is known apart from his writings, was another anatomist who engaged Rymsdyk to depict his specimens. Jenty came to London about 1745, and taught anatomy and surgery. His two publications with which Rymsdyk was associated were first published in 1757, and each had an octavo text volume accompanying the folio plates. The anatomical tables were advertised in 1756 and published in the following year as *An essay on the demonstration of the human structure, half as large as nature, in four tables, from the pictures painted after dissections, for that purpose*, London, 1757. The plates were drawn by Rymsdyk and engraved by Edward Fisher, two being dated 1756. Jenty's *the demonstrations of a pregnant uterus of a woman at her full term. In six tables, as large as nature. Done from pictures painted after dissections, by Mr. Riemsdyk*, was also published by the author from his own house in 1757, and was re-issued in the following year. The plates were intended to be coloured, but probably the cost of the process decided Jenty against this (Plate 33). In a note to the reader, Jenty explains why mezzotint was chosen:

> "If it should be asked, Why, in these Plates, I chose Mezzotinto, instead of Engraving? I answer, that not only the difficulty and Length of time requisite to have executed these TABLES, by able persons, nor the expence, which would have been considerable, prevented my Determination to Engraving; but the Engraving itself, how well soever performed, would not have answered my intention for Colouring, so well as Mezzotinto; as this method is softer, and capable of exhibiting a nearer imitation of Nature than Engraving, as Artists themselves acknowledge that Nature may admit of light and shades, well blended and softened, but never did of a harsh outline: So it must be confessed, that these Prints may want the Smartness which Engraving might have contributed; but the Softness which they possess, may approach nearer to the Imitation of Nature, when coloured, than any engraving possibly could, merely thro' the unavoidable Delineation of the Outline.
>
> Gentlemen may have these Mezzotinto Prints, coloured after the original Pictures, of different Degrees of Perfection, according to the Price allowed to the Colourer."

There were Latin, German and Dutch translations with mezzotint plates, but the French version had both text and plates engraved. (See De Lint, 1916; and Thornton and Want, 1978).

Rymsdyk made numerous drawings for Jenty between 1755 and 1757, though not all were used in his two atlases. In 1757 Jenty presented to the Company of Surgeons "four large anatomical prints, coloured, glazed and framed", but these have not been traced. It appears that Jenty disposed of much of his property before joining the British Expeditionary Force in 1762, and John Fothergill (1712-1780) acquired Rymsdyk's original coloured crayon drawings, which he sent as a gift to Pennsylvania Hospital via William Shippen (1736-1808). These drawings, still in Pennsylvania Hospital, played an important part in early medical education in the United States. They consisted of eighteen drawings framed and glazed, of which one was by Thomas Burgess, and sixteen by Rymsdyk, the other being a picture of a doctor feeling the pulse. They include the originals used for the reproductions in Jenty's two atlases, although there are certain differences between the originals and the mezzotints. The

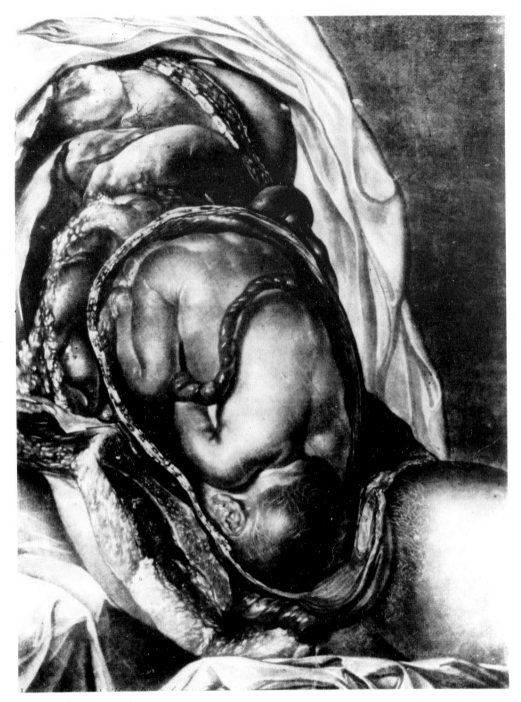

Plate 33. Mezzotint of Rymsdyk's drawing of the pregnant uterus at term, from C.N. Jenty's *Demonstrations of a pregnant uterus*, London, 1757.

drawings in the Pennsylvania Hospital have been described by J. A. Scott (1904), four of them being reproduced in colour by Greim (1952), and all were reproduced in an article by Edward B. Krumbhaar (1922).

It would appear that Rymsdyk's first drawings after his appearance in London in 1750 were executed for William Hunter, and were eventually to be published in Hunter's *Gravid uterus* in 1774. In fact, Rymsdyk's final drawing for this was made in 1772, so that he had been working for Hunter on this subject for twenty-two years. William Hunter (1718-1783) had gone to London in 1741, after studying in Glasgow and Edinburgh. He resided with Smellie for a few weeks, then went to live with James Douglas (1675-1742) as assistant, and as tutor to his son. William Hunter derived great benefit from his friendship with both these distinguished fellow-Scots, and was greatly influenced by them during his early years in London. Douglas died in 1742, but William Hunter continued to live in the Douglas household, and to benefit from the extensive collection of manuscripts and drawings left by Douglas. William Hunter was admitted a member of the Corporation of Surgeons in 1747, and then became "surgeon accoucheur" to Middlesex Hospital and to the British Lying-in Hospital. He obtained a Glasgow M.D. in 1750, and a few years later he left the Corporation of Surgeons and was admitted as a licentiate of the College of Physicians in 1756. This transfer from the practice of "surgeon accoucheur" to "physician accoucheur" was important at that time, as physicians were regarded as better-educated than surgeons, who had served apprenticeships rather than attended universities. This difference in social standing resulted in physicians becoming more opulent than surgeons, and although both operated as men-midwives, the physicians had more successful practices, attending women of the upper classes rather than the poor. William Smellie worked among the poor, whereas William Hunter attended Queen Charlotte, and was appointed her Physician-Extraordinary. He acquired wealth which enabled him to build up remarkable collections of pictures, books, manuscripts, coins, medals and other objects which he left to Glasgow University.

William Hunter was a perfectionist, and when he planned his atlas illustrating the gravid uterus he engaged Rymsdyk to make the drawings, Robert Strange to supervise the engraving of the plates, two of which Strange himself engraved, and eventually Hunter chose John Baskerville to print the book. Initially, Hunter had intended to publish ten plates of the gravid uterus at term, and the plates were prepared, but a second, and then a third subject being available in various stages of gestation, Hunter decided to present an entire series showing the principal changes which occur during the nine months of utero-gestation. He had advertised the first set of drawings as early as October 1751, but there were many delays in obtaining suitable subjects for dissection, and it was 1772 before Rymsdyk made his final drawing for the atlas. There are sixty-one drawings made by him for the *Anatomy of the gravid uterus*, preserved in the Hunterian Collection at Glasgow, and most of these are featured in the thirty-one plates of the thirty-four contained in the atlas. Three of the plates were from drawings by other artists: Plate XVI was drawn by Edward Edwards (1738-1806); Plate XXI was drawn by Alexander Cozens (c. 1717-1786); and Plate XXII was drawn by Nicholas Blakey (d. 1758). Plate XXXII was the only one engraved by Rymsdyk, but there were at least sixteen engravers engaged in the preparation of the copper-plates. Charles Grignion (1717-1810), who had engraved the plates for Smellie, engraved Plate VIII, and (Sir) Robert Strange (1721-1792) engraved Plates IV (Plate 34) and V. Strange was a great friend of William Hunter: in addition to advising him on the

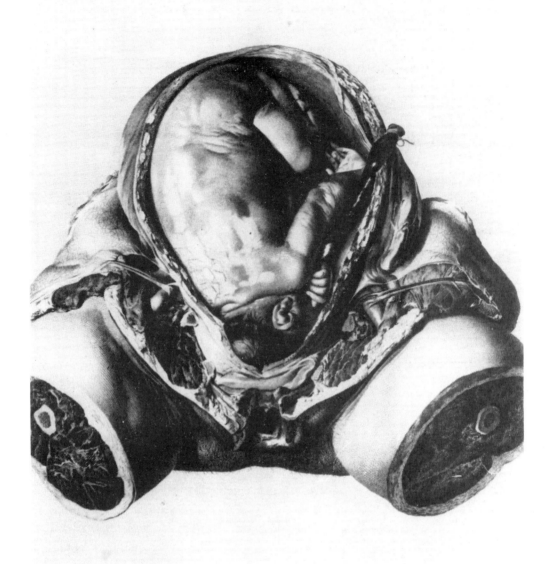

Plate 34. Engraving by Robert Strange of Rymsdyk's drawing for William Hunter's *Gravid uterus*, Birmingham, 1774.

purchase of pictures, he supervised the engraving of the plates. Hunter praised him in his introduction with the words:

> "He owes likewise much to the ingenious artists who made the drawings and engravings; and particularly to Mr. Strange, not only for having by his own hand secured a sort of immortality to two of his plates, but for having given his advice and assistance in every part with a steady and disinterested friendship."

The name "Rymsdyk" is not mentioned, although he was responsible for most of the original drawings!

Hunter had at one time intended to publish the book from a press to be installed on his own premises, but he obviously encountered difficulties. It was to be elephant folio in size, with the best paper, ink and type used both for plates and text. He was acquainted with the books already published by John Baskerville (1706-1775) of Birmingham, and decided that his requirements could best be met by that first-class craftsman. His atlas was finally published as *The anatomy of the human gravid uterus exhibited in figures*, printed in Birmingham by John Baskerville, 1774, with pages originally measuring 22 x 16½ inches. The title-page contains the details printed in both Latin and English, and the textual descriptions opposite the plates are also in both languages. It was the most sumptuous medical publication of the eighteenth century, and obviously cost Hunter vast sums of money, which he could not hope to recoup. He had intended to supplement the atlas by publishing a separate text on the anatomy of the gravid uterus, but he left the manuscript for this uncompleted at his death. It was published twenty years after the atlas as *An anatomical description of the human gravid uterus and its contents*, London, 1794, being edited by his nephew, Matthew Baillie, with a second edition by Edward Rigby published in 1843. Rymsdyk made many other drawings for William Hunter during this period, most of which were not published. They are preserved in the Hunterian Collection, Glasgow, and further information on these, on the drawings in the *Gravid uterus*, and on the authors of the other books illustrated by Rymsdyk is contained in Thornton and Want (1974 a-b); Ollerenshaw (1974); and Thornton (1982).

When Rymsdyk had finished working for William Hunter he began work on the preparation of his own publication, the *Museum Britannicum*. Obtaining permission to make drawings of objects in the newly-opened British Museum, he and his son Andrew Van Rymsdyk produced a miscellany of drawings for the book, which was an unofficial guide to the collection. Jan Van Rymsdyk was responsible for the text and twenty of the plates, Andrew contributing drawings for the other twelve. The book was produced as a folio in 1778, and the text reveals something of Jan Van Rymsdyk's early life, expressing his emotions as a frustrated portrait painter forced to earn his living as a medical artist. Attacking the attitude of society to his fellow-artists, he reviled authors, engravers, and many other professional men, and singled out William Hunter in the guise of "Dr. Ibis". He resented the fact that Hunter appears to have made no effort to further Rymsdyk's ambitions as a portrait painter, and also that his work for Hunter had not, to his mind, received adequate recognition. Rymsdyk stated that he had made his last medical drawing, but circumstances decided otherwise.

Possibly the *Museum Britannicum* was not as successful as Jan Van Rymsdyk had anticipated. He had certainly spent several years in preparing it, and a great deal of money on the employment of engravers, and on having the book printed. It contains a curious conglomeration of miscellaneous engravings of unconnected objects, and the text, although revealing more about Rymsdyk than can be gleaned elsewhere, cannot have endeared him to his readers. The original drawings are now housed in the British Museum, Department of Prints and Drawings, and have been described by J. L. Thornton (1982).

It would appear that Jan Van Rymsdyk found that he still had to earn a living, but his book had probably made it impossible for him to expect his former patrons, John and William Hunter, to employ him as an artist. Rymsdyk seemed to have disappeared from the London scene after the publication of his book, but he reappeared about 1783 making drawings for Thomas Denman (1733-1815). William Hunter died in that year, and was succeeded as London's leading obstetrician by Denman. Among several other publications, Denman was the author of *A collection of engravings, tending to illustrate the generation and parturition of animals, and the human species*, a folio published in 1787. In his preface Denman states:

> "Some years ago, without any view to this publication, I began to have drawings taken of such subjects as occurred to me relative to utero-gestation or parturition in the human species, or in animals, natural, preternatural, or morbid; whenever they appeared likely to give a more comprehensive view of the science of Midwifery, or to improve the art; . . . and there is so much truth and elegance in the drawings executed by Mr. Rymsdyk they may be considered as patterns for all future artists. Some of these being engraved, I am unwilling that they should be lost, and therefore publish this first number as a specimen of the work."

The *Collection* consists of nine plates, six of which were engraved from original drawings by Rymsdyk, these bearing various dates of publication between 22 December 1783 and 23 February 1787. One drawing by Rymsdyk is dated 1784 by him, and is of the human uterus at term, a subject Rymsdyk had depicted for William Hunter in 1750, William Smellie in 1751, and C. N. Jenty in 1757. (See Thornton and Want, 1979). All the illustrations in the *Collection* were included in the third, 1801, edition of Denman's *Introduction to the practice of midwifery*, together with other plates, one of which was drawn by Rymsdyk. The plates were also issued separately in *Engravings, representing the generation of some animals; some circumstances attending parturition in the human species; and a few of the diseases to which the sex is liable*, a quarto volume published in 1815. Most of the plates had previously been published, but Plate IV is of particular interest because it was drawn by "J V. Rymsdyk" and the date of publication is given as 23 February 1789, twelve years before its first appearance in Denman's *Introduction* (1801), and two years after his *Collection of engravings* had been published, suggesting that it was probably drawn in 1788, as all the additional plates are dated between 1788 and 1801. This is the last reference to Jan Van Rymsdyk we have traced, and he probably died in either 1788 or 1789, disappearing as mysteriously as he had appeared in London in 1750.

The outstanding anatomist of his period, Giovanni Domenico Santorini (1681-1737), was educated at Bologna, Padua and Pisa before teaching anatomy in Venice, where he became physician to the Spandaletto of the city. Santorini dissected and drew the gross features of the body, including the facial muscles involved in the expression of the emotions. He was the author of the

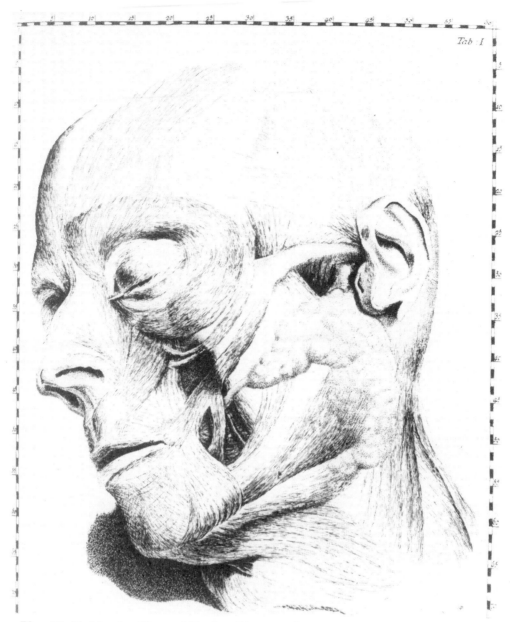

Plate 35. Etching by Giovanni Battista Piazzetta, from Giovanni Domenico Santorini:
Septemdecim tabulas quas nunc primum edit atque explicat, Parma, 1775.

posthumously-published *Septemdecim tabulas quas nunc primum edit atque explicat iisque alias addit de structura mammarum et de tunica testis vaginali Michael Girardi*, Parma, 1775, a folio containing forty-two engraved plates, of which twenty-one are in outline with reference letters. The copper-plates are in a light crayon effect, similar to etchings. Seventeen of the Santorini plates have ruled margins, and were drawn by Giovanni Battista Piazzetta (1682-1754). They had been engraved by a woman, Florentia Marcella, under the personal supervision of Santorini (Plate 35). Two other plates belonged to Giovanni Battista Covoli (died 1768), and two to Michele Girardi (1731-1797), these being drawn by Ignazio Gasparotti and engraved by Giuseppe Patrini (1711-1786).

Samuel Thomas von Soemmerring (1755-1830), who employed and trained Christian Köck to draw the illustrations for his books, was himself an artist of no mean ability. He admired the work of Albinus, and followed him in his aim for both artistic and scientific accuracy. Soemmerring was born in Thorn and studied at Göttingen before visiting England, Scotland and the Netherlands, meeting William Hunter and Pieter Camper on his travels. In 1779 he became professor of anatomy in Cassel, and later established himself as a physician in Frankfurt-on-Main. Köck, who died in 1818, lived with Soemmerring for many years, although he once left his patron to go to Moscow, and Soemmerring had great difficulty in securing his return. Köck drew innumerable illustrations for Soemmerring, many of which were not published until they appeared in his posthumous works. His literary output was prodigious, and the following are particularly noteworthy for their illustrations.

His inaugural dissertation, *De basi encephali et originibus nervorum cranio egredientium*, Göttingen, 1778, contains four plates in quarto drawn by Soemmerring and engraved by Carl Christian Glassbach, Jr. They show a cross-section of the brain, with its base and the relevant nerves. *Über die Wirkungen der Schnürbrüste*, Berlin, 1793, is a second edition of his work illustrating the disfigurement caused by wearing tightly-laced corsets, but only the second issue contains the plate. This copper-plate in oblong folio was drawn by Christian Köck and engraved by Daniel Berger.

Soemmerring set out to represent the most perfect and faithful representation of the female skeleton to accompany that of a male skeleton published by Albinus. The resultant *Tabula sceleti femini juncta descriptione*, Frankfurt-on-Main, 1797, contains Köck's drawing of the idealized female skeleton, which was engraved in Stuttgart by Baehrenstecher under the direction of Johann Gotthard von Müller.

William Hunter's *The anatomy of the human gravid uterus*, 1774, did not deal in detail with the early development of the embryo, and Soemmerring planned to remedy this in his *Icones embryonum humanorum*, Frankfurt-on-Main, 1799. This contains two large folio copper-plates and two vignettes, drawn by Christian Köck, and engraved by F. L. Neubauer, Hüllmann, and the Klauber brothers. In the same year appeared *Tabula baseos encephali*, Frankfurt-on-Main, 1799, with two plates drawn by Köck and engraved by Pierre Michel Alix (born 1752). A survey of the history of the study of the fetus has been made by B. A. Salvadori (1981) in a well-illustrated article containing an extensive bibliography of the subject.

Described by Choulant (1945, p. 308) as "Soemmerring's most perfect work", *Abbildungen des menschlichen Auges*, Frankfurt-on-Main, 1801, became "the foundation for all modern researches on the structure of this organ". It contains sixteen copper-plates, some of which are coloured, Christian Köck having made the drawings, which were engraved by Vincenzo Scarpati, the brothers Klauber, Clemens Koll (1754-1807), Johann Christoph Bock (born 1752), and Johann Conrad Felsing (1766-1819).

These are only a selection of the outstanding publications by Soemmerring, and indicate his wide interests, which continued to be displayed long after his

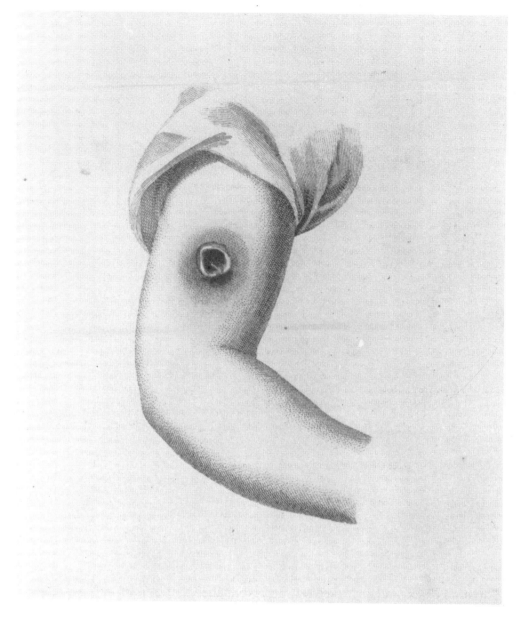

Plate 36. Drawing by Edward Pearce, engraved by William Skelton, to illustrate Edward Jenner's *An inquiry into the causes and effects of the variolae vaccinae*, London, 1798.

death in 1830. The plates inspired by him influenced future authors and artists by their accuracy and beauty, and they retain an important position in the history of medical illustration.

One other book published towards the end of the eighteenth century must be mentioned both for its significance in the history of medicine, and for its illustrations, which have frequently been reproduced, and emphasize the value of simple drawings to demonstrate technical descriptions. Edward Jenner (1749-1823), a native of Berkeley, Gloucestershire, where he spent most of his life, was a pupil of John Hunter, and shared his keen interest in natural history.

95

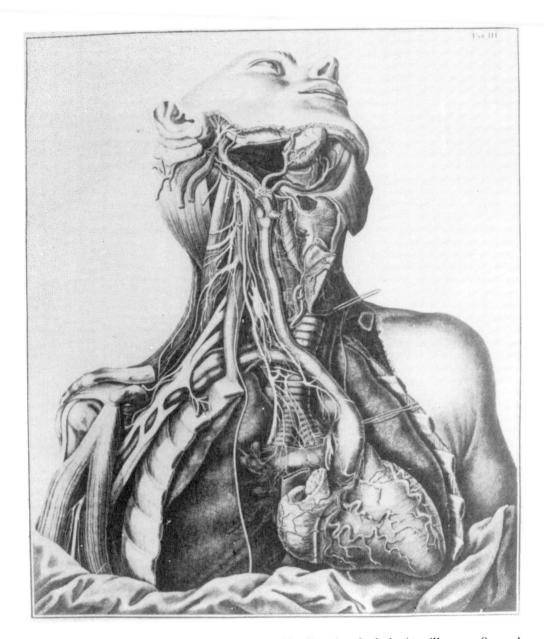

Plate 37. Drawing by Antonio Scarpa, engraved by Faustino Anderloni, to illustrate Scarpa's
Tabulae neurologicae ad illustrandam historiam cardiacorum, Pavia, 1794.

His claim to fame in medicine rests, however, in his pioneer experiments with
vaccination, first made in 1796. Jenner's pamphlet on the subject was printed
for the author by Sampson Low with the title *An inquiry into the causes and
effects of the variolae vaccinae, a disease discovered in some of the western
counties of England, particularly Gloucestershire, and known by the name of the
cow pox*, London, 1798. A quarto of seventy-five pages, it contains four coloured
plates (Plate 36), the first of which was drawn and engraved by William Skelton,
the others being drawn by Edward Pearce, and engraved by Skelton. The plates
were hand-coloured, and in the second edition they were coloured by W. Cuff.

William R. LeFanu (1951) has provided full information on this classic publication, and on Jenner's other books, articles and manuscripts, in *A bio-bibliography of Edward Jenner 1749-1823*.

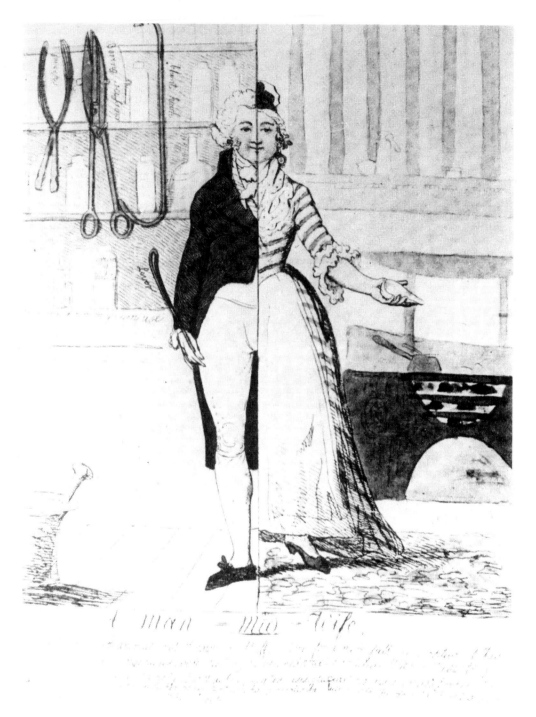

Plate 38. Use of caricature in medical book illustration in S.W. Fores: *Man-midwifery dissected: or, the obstetric family instructor*, London, 1796.

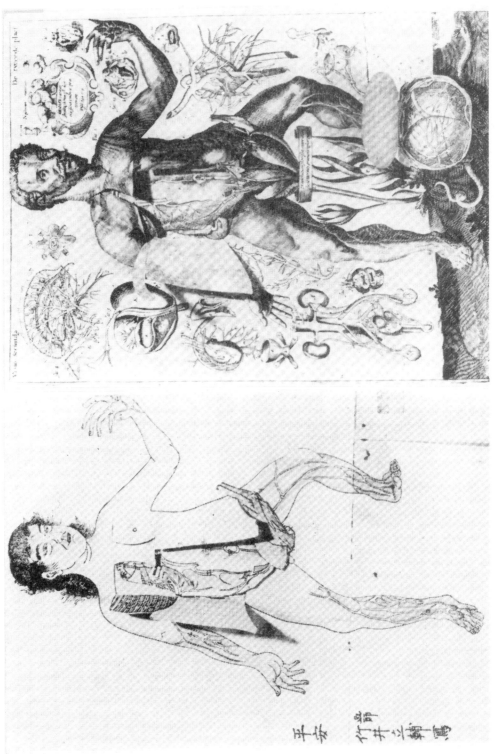

Plate 39. Japanese adaptation of a figure from Johann Remmelin, derived from a Dutch translation published in Amsterdam, 1667.

Antonio Scarpa (1752-1832) was appointed professor of anatomy at Modena in 1772, and visited England in 1780, when he met Percivall Pott, William and John Hunter, and William Cruikshank. He became professor of anatomy at Padua, where he had been educated, in 1783. Scarpa illustrated his own writings, the plates being engraved by Faustino Anderloni (1766-1847), who had been trained by Scarpa. W. J. Bishop (1954) states that John Bostock (1773-1846) described these engravings as "admirably expressive of the subject, without the gaudiness of the French engravers, who appear to aim principally at effect, or the tameness of the English, who seem to think of little except economy". Scarpa was the author of several significant books, which went into numerous editions and translations, but his outstanding contribution was *Tabulae neurologicae ad illustrandam historiam caridacorum*, Pavia, 1794, which describes and demonstrates the nerves of the heart (Plate 37). He also made important observations on aneurysm, hernia, the ear and diseases of the eye. His keen interest in art also resulted in the formation of a large art collection.

An early example of the use of caricature in medical book illustration was included in *Man-midwifery dissected: or, the obstetric family instructor*, London, 1793, printed for the author S. W. Fores writing under the pseudonym "John Blunt". The folding frontispiece, coloured in the original, is here reproduced as Plate 38.

Traditional medicine was practised in Japan until Western medicine was introduced towards the middle of the sixteenth century. The Netherlands East Indies Company was founded in 1602, and Dutch influence dominated all western learning filtering into Japan. Japanese physicians were personally instructed by Dutch physicians. The *Kaitai shinsho* appears to be the first medical publication in Japanese, and was issued in five volumes in 1774. The original of this in Dutch, itself a translation of a German work by Johann Adam Kulmus, was published in Danzig in 1722 with the title *Anatomische Tabellen*. The illustrations in the Japanese version are inferior to those in the original, but *Kaitai shinsho* greatly influenced the development of modern medical practice in Japan by introducing the basic principles of anatomy. Ranzaburō Ōtori (1964) has provided additional information on the introduction of Western medicine into Japan, and an example of Japanese adaptation of a figure from a book originally by Johann Remmelin is featured here in Plate 39. This was derived from a Dutch translation of Remmelin, published in Amsterdam in 1667.

CHAPTER 7

THE NINETEENTH CENTURY

"Art has become more and more indispensable to us as an aid both to record and to explication. The diagram, the more highly finished drawing, the photograph, and the model, serve as a new language that speaks with strength and clearness where written or spoken words would convey their meaning slowly and imperfectly."

William Anderson (1886).

One of the most important innovations affecting medical illustration in the nineteenth century was the introduction of lithography. This differs from processes used earlier in the fact that the plate is neither carved in relief nor incised. The design to be printed is drawn directly onto a flat piece of stone or metal with a specially-prepared greasy chalk pencil. The surface is then soaked with water. This is absorbed except by the greased sections, and when printing ink is applied it is accepted by the greasy areas, but rejected by the wetted portions. Lithography was invented by Alois Senefelder (1771-1834) in 1796, and the original stone used was known as "Pierre de Bavière". Senefelder patented his discovery in London as "polyautography" in 1801. It was renamed "lithographie" in France in 1803. Senefelder remained in London for only seven months, and sold his patent to Philip André for three thousand pounds, but the process did not initially become popular in England. Senefelder's successors followed him back to the Continent, where the art was developed in France, Germany and Austria. Johann Anton André and his family were among those who improved upon the art, and their efforts were recorded in a book written in German by Senefelder, and translated into French a few years later as *L'Art de la lithographie, ou instruction practique containent la description claire et succinte des differens procédés à suivre pour dessiner, graver et imprimer sur pierre; précedée d'une histoire de la lithographie et de ses divers progrès*, Paris, 1819. This records the invention of the lithographic process, and the improvements effected in the technique over a period of twenty years. It also contains a portrait of the author, a lithographed title-page, and nineteen other full-page lithographs.

Matthew Baillie (1761-1823), the "father of medical pathology", was the nephew of William and John Hunter, and lived with William after spending five years at Glasgow University. Baillie was the main beneficiary in William Hunter's will, and succeeded him at the Great Windmill Street School. William's museum was the main source of the illustrations for Matthew Baillie's most famous work, *The morbid anatomy of some of the most important parts of the human body*, London, 1783, the plates for which were published

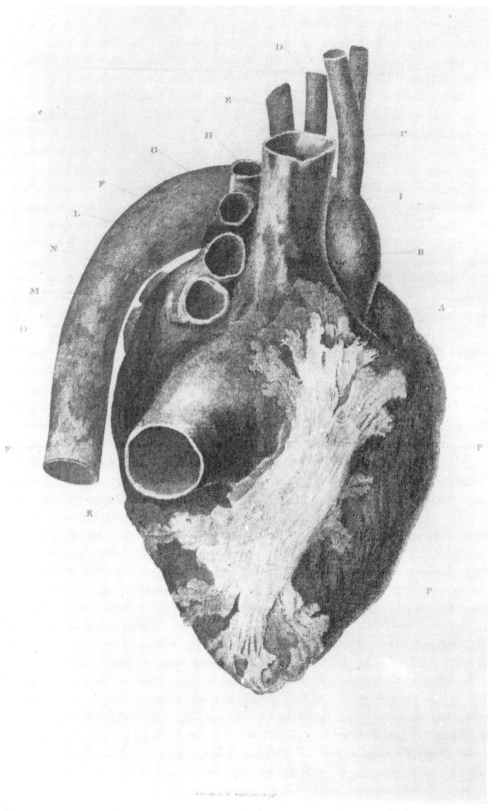

Plate 40. Engraving of a drawing by William Clift to illustrate Matthew Baillie's *The morbid anatomy of some of the most important parts of the human body*, London, 1783. The plates were issued in book form in 1803.

separately in ten fasciculi between 1799 and 1802, and issued in book form in 1803 as *A series of engravings, accompanied with explanations, which are intended to ilustrate the morbid anatomy of some of the most important parts of the human body*, London (Plate 40). William Clift (1775-1849) made the original drawings for these illustrations, working for almost two years on their preparation, and he was paid one guinea for each drawing. Twenty-four of the originals are in the Royal College of Physicians of London, and the remaining forty-eight are in the Medical Library of the University of Melbourne. Harold D. Attwood (private communication, 11 February 1982) informs us that it is hoped to publish a facsimile of Baillie's *Engravings* from the copy which probably belonged to William Clift, together with his original drawings which are contained in that copy. Incidentally, the engravers received five guineas for each of the plates, which probably reflects the difference between the value placed on the work of the respective professions. Clift came to London from Bodmin in 1792 as amanuensis to John Hunter and, after Hunter's death, Clift continued to look after Hunter's museum, eventually to become Conservator, and a Fellow of the Royal Society. His remarkable career has been the subject of a biography by Jessie Dobson (1954). He arrived in London with artistic ability, which he extended and exploited for the benefit of John Hunter's collection, and for many others. He also made drawings for Everard Home, William Long, Astley Cooper, Nathaniel Highmore, William Buckland, among others, and his work was used to illustrate some of their publications. William LeFanu (1971) has provided further information on Clift's work, and some of his drawings, and his diaries, are preserved in the Royal College of Surgeons Library.

Both John Bell (1763-1820) and his brother Sir Charles Bell (1774-1842) of Edinburgh were outstanding artists as well as leading surgeons and anatomists. They were authors of numerous books, most of which went into many editions and translations, the majority of the illustrations having been drawn, and sometimes engraved by Sir Charles. John Bell was a founder of vascular surgery, and was the author of, among other books, *Anatomy of the bones, muscles and joints*, two volumes, Edinburgh, [1793]-1797, which was re-issued in four volumes, 1797-1804; *Engravings explaining the anatomy of the bones, muscles and joints*, Edinburgh, three volumes, (vol. 1, Edinburgh; vols. 2-3 London), 1794-1804, the third volume of which was almost entirely the work of his brother Charles; and *Principles of surgery*, three volumes (in four), 1801-1808, which is particularly valued for its engravings and historical material.

Sir Charles Bell was the author of *A system of dissections*, two volumes, Edinburgh, 1798-1803; and *Engravings of the arteries*, London, 1801, the illustrations in which were also engraved by Bell. His original twelve water-colours and copper-plate writing for this book, preserved in a small volume in the National Library of Medicine, Washington, have been reproduced in black-and-white by Harold Wellington Jones (1937). These books were followed by *The anatomy of the brain explained in a series of engravings*, London, 1802, containing twelve coloured plates; *A series of engravings explaining the course of the nerves*, London, 1803; *Essays on the anatomy of expression in painting*, 1806, second edition, 1824 (Plate 41); *A system of operative surgery*, two volumes,

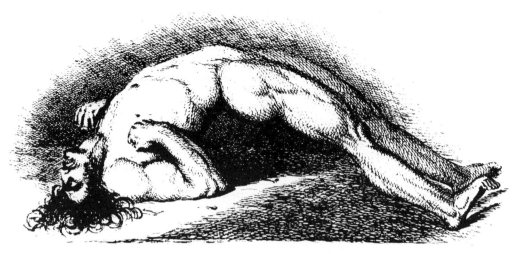

Plate 41. Illustration of opisthotonus made by Sir Charles Bell for his *The anatomy of expression*, 2nd ed., London, 1824.

London, 1807-1809; *Idea of a new anatomy of the brain*, which was first privately printed in London in 1811, and expounds Bell's law based on the discovery of one-way traffic in nerves; *Illustrations of the great operations of surgery*, London, 1821; and *The nervous system of the human body*, London 1830, which includes descriptions of "Bell's nerve", and "Bell's palsy". A Bridgewater treatise by Bell was published by William Pickering with the title *The hand, its mechanism and vital endowments as evidencing design*, 1833; this contains three engravings which were copied without acknowledgement from Cheselden's *Osteographia*, 1733 (LeFanu, 1961). Sir Charles Bell was the author of several other books and articles, details of which are included in an extensive biographical study by Sir Gordon Gordon-Taylor and E. W. Walls (1958).

Three processes were employed in the reproduction of the illustrations in *The morbid anatomy of the human uterus and its appendages*, London, 1832, by Richard Hooper (1773-1835). The plates were drawn by J. Howship, and the aquatints by T. Heaphy are a close approximation to water-colour painting. Heaphy was also responsible for the lithographs, and these and the stipple engravings were also reproduced in colour. A black-and-white photograph of an aquatint (Plate 42) can give some idea of the details in the plates, but the originals must be seen for their delicacy and colouring to be fully appreciated. Robert Hooper was a successful physician, and lectured to large classes in Savile Road, London. He was particularly interested in pathological anatomy, amassing a valuable collection of specimens, on which his publications were based. The plates in his *Morbid anatomy* bear various dates, and might have been issued separately before being collected together in the book.

The first anatomical atlas to be illustrated with lithographs was the magnificent folio by Jules Germain Cloquet (1790-1883), published in Paris with the title *Anatomie de l'homme, ou description et figures lithographiées de toutes les parties du corps humain* (Plate 43). The 300 plates were published in fifty-one sections over the ten-year period between 1821 and 1831, and the

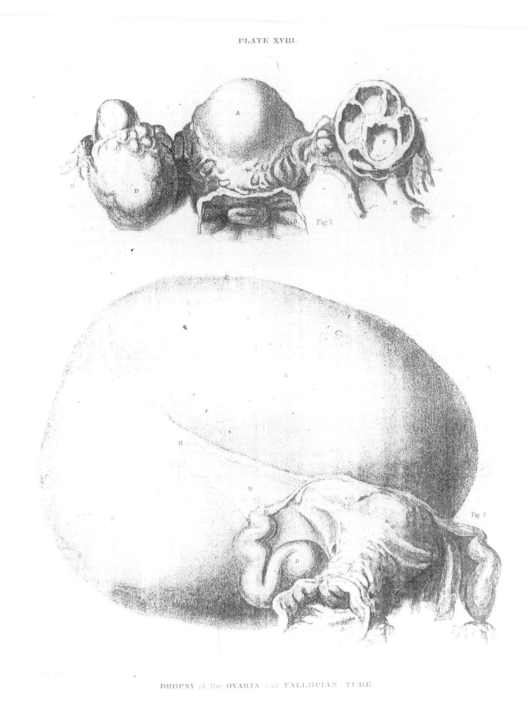

Plate 42. Aquatint by T. Heaphy of drawing by J. Howship, from Richard Hooper: *The morbid anatomy of the human uterus and its appendages*, London, 1832.

lithographs were printed in the two first ateliers of Paris, both of which were founded in 1816. They were established by Charles de Lasteyrie and Godefroy Engelmann, who were among the pioneers of the development of the lithographic art in France. Another monumental anatomical atlas was published over a period of thirteen years in forty folio sections, to form two volumes when bound. This was *Anatomie pathologique du corps humain, ou*

104

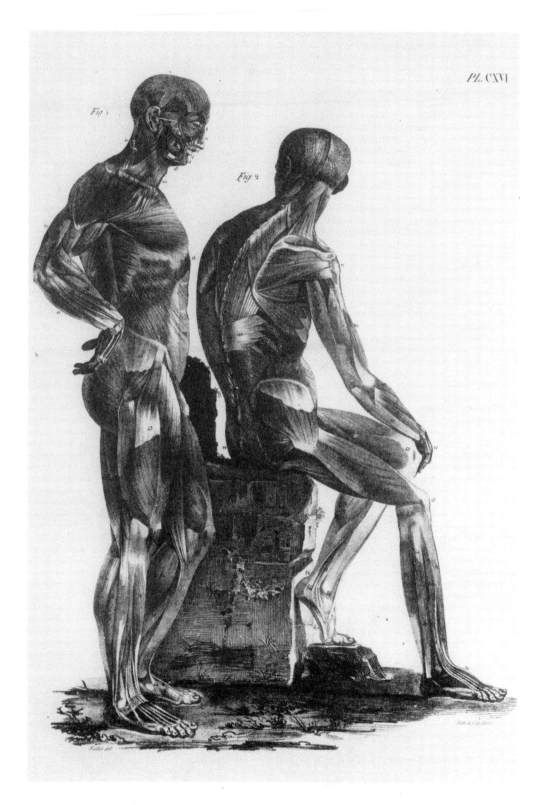

Plate 43. Lithograph by Charles de Lasteyrie, from Jules Germain Cloquet's *Anatomie de l'homme*, Paris, 1821-1831.

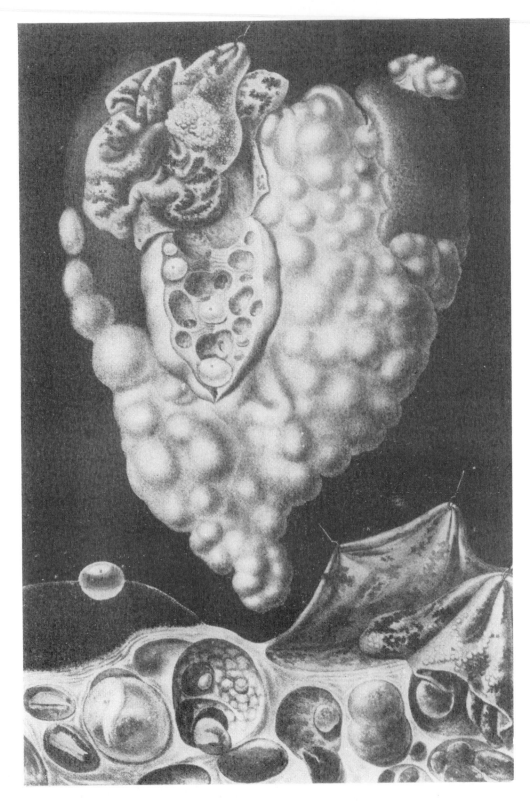

Plate 44. Lithograph by Antoine Chazel, from Jean Creuveilhier's *Anatomie pathologique du corps humain*, Paris, 1829-1842.

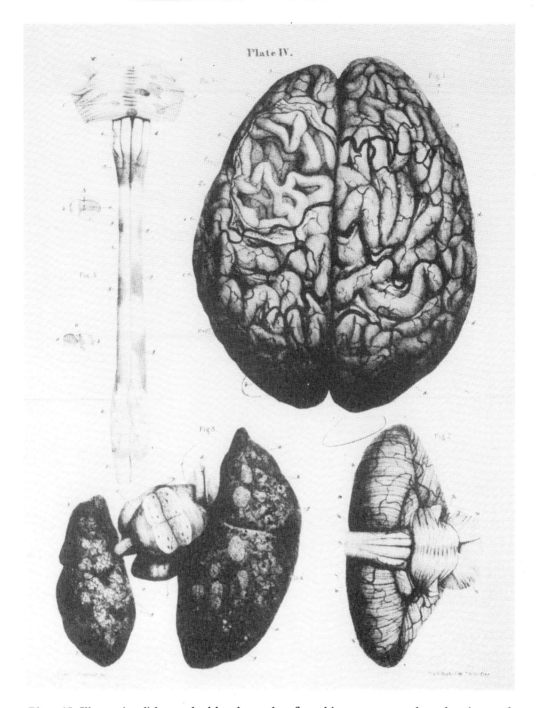

Plate 45. Illustration lithographed by the author from his own water-colour drawing, and published in Sir Robert Carswell's *Pathological anatomy*, London, 1838.

descriptions, avec figures lithographiées et coloriées, des divers altérations morbides dont le corps humain est susceptible, by Jean Creuveilhier (1781-1874), and published in Paris by J. B. Baillière between 1829 and 1842. This contains 233 full-page lithographic plates, most of which were the work of Antoine Chazel (Plate 44). Yet another outstanding folio containing coloured lithographs is notable for the fact that the plates were drawn on stone by the author,

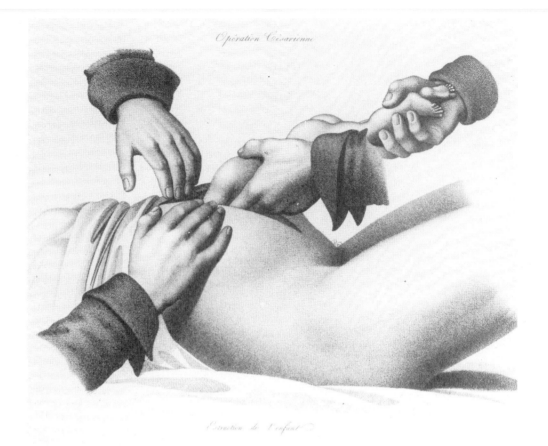

Plate 46. Drawing by Antoine Chazel, engraved by Forestier and Couché fils, from Jacques Pierre Maygrier's *Nouvelles démonstrations d'accouchemens*, Paris, 1822-1827.

Sir Robert Carswell (1793-1857), a native of Paisley who became professor of morbid anatomy at University College, London, in 1828. He made 2000 water-colour drawings of pathological specimens, and produced the folio of 48 hand-coloured plates which was published as *Pathological anatomy. Illustrations of the elementary forms of disease*, London, 1838 (Plate 45).

Jacques Pierre Maygrier (1771-1835) was an army surgeon who later went to Paris to study anatomy and obstetrics, becoming a pupil of Antoine Dubois, accoucheur to the Empress Marie Louise. Maygrier built up an extensive obstetric practice, and his book on the subject was issued over a period of five years in twenty parts, with a large folding plate and 79 full-page engravings. The text is greatly enhanced by the splendid illustrations, which were executed with utmost accuracy. Entitled *Nouvelles démonstrations d'accouchemens*, Paris, 1822-(1827), many copies are not complete, as so often happens in books which have been issued in parts. The drawings were executed by Antoine Chazel, and were engraved by Forestier and Couché fils, who produced an interesting stipple effect such as in that showing the extraction of the child in Caesarean section (Plate 46).

John James Pringle (1855-1925) edited the *Pictorial atlas of the skin diseases and syphilitic affections . . . from models in the Museum of the Saint-Louis*

Hospital, London, 1897, which was published by the Rebman Publishing Company. The fifty full-page colour photolithographs were made from wax models, and represent the value of the combination of the techniques of the artist using wax as his medium, and the use of colour photography printed on a lithographic plate (Plate 47). Dermatology is a particularly difficult subject to illustrate, colour being of vital importance in the specific identification of diseases of the skin. Black-and-white illustrations of skin conditions are of little value in textbooks, and the development of both colour photography and improved methods of colour reproduction, have enhanced the value of illustrations in dermatological literature. Unfortunately, exact colour reproduction remains an expensive process.

Obviously, many other important illustrated medical books were published during the nineteenth-century, and the above has been selected as representative of various techniques and subjects, as well as for their historical significance. Fielding Hudson Garrison wrote a section on "Anatomical illustration since the time of Choulant" for the 1917 edition of Choulant's book, which appears as Appendix III in Choulant (1945, pp. 403-412). This contains lists of illustrated treatises on anatomy, with some information on the methods of illustration, and the artists involved. The outstanding anatomical atlases are recorded, and we note the development of modern scientific medicine from the middle of the nineteenth century. We see the development of direct photography for medical illustration, of lithography, electroplating, zincography and other reproductive processes, but also a revival of wood-engraving. The elephant folios of the previous century were no longer evident, and copper, steel and mezzotint engravings had almost disappeared from the medical scene.

One of the most outstanding anatomical treatises of the period was the three-volume *Handbuch der systematischen Anatomie des Menschen* by Jacob Henle (1809-1885), published in Braunschweig, 1856-1873, which was illustrated by the author in his "architectural drawing" method which demonstrates cross-sections of structure through different axes and planes. This was followed by his *Anatomischer Hand-Atlas zum Gebrauch im Secirsaal*, published in six parts between 1871 and 1876. Another textbook written for students, illustrated in a similar manner, was *An elementary treatise on human anatomy*, by Joseph Leidy (1823-1891), published in Philadelphia in 1861, with a second edition in 1889. Joseph Hyrtl (1811-1894) was the author of *Die Corrosions-Anatomie und ihre Ergebnisse*, Vienna, 1873, containing lithographs from drawings made by C. Heitzmann. Life-size superimposed plates were included in *Anatomie iconoclastique. Atlas complémentaire de tous les ouvrages traitant de l'anatomie et de la physiologie humaines, composé de planches découpées, coloriées et superposées*, by Gustave Jules A. Witkowski (born 1843) and published in twelve parts, Paris, 1874-1888. Superimposed plates were also incorporated in two books by Etienne Rabaud (born 1868), *Anatomie élémentaire du corps humain*, Paris, 1899, and *Atlas anatomique du corps de l'homme et de la femme*, Paris, 1905.

Carl Gegenbaur (1826-1903) was the author of *Lehrbuch der Anatomie des Menschen*, Leipzig, 1883, which contains 558 partly coloured woodcuts; 750 partly-coloured lithographs are an important feature in the *Handatlas der*

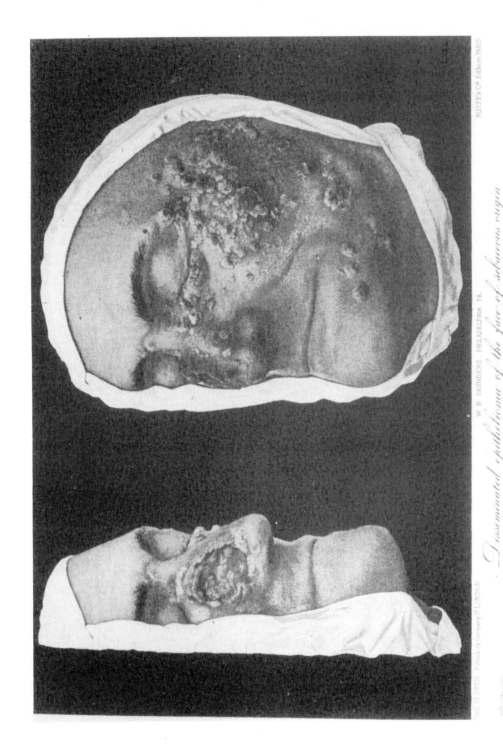

Plate 47. Colour photolithograph made from wax model, from John James Pringle's *Pictorial atlas of the skin diseases,*
London, 1897.

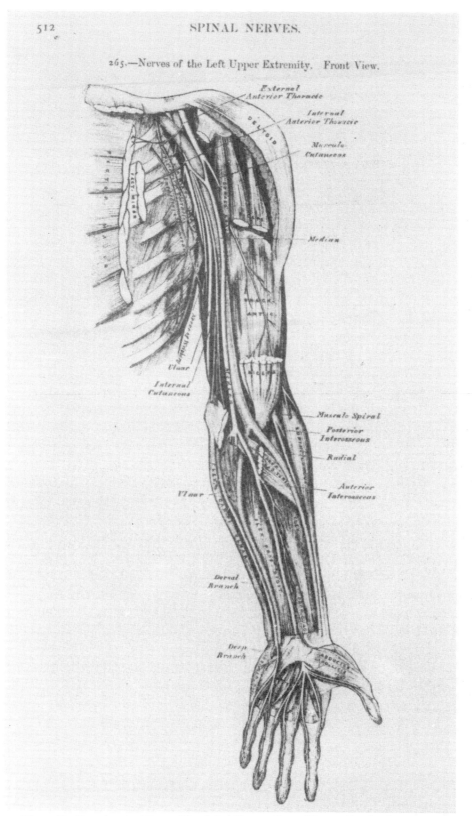

Plate 48. Drawing by Henry Vandyke Carter, from Henry Gray's *Anatomy*, London, 1858.

Anatomie des Menschen of Karl Werner Spalteholz, published in three volumes, Leipzig, 1895-1903, which was translated into English by Lewellys F. Barker, 1900-1903, and which is still maintained up-to-date as a useful anatomical atlas for students. German and French systems of anatomy are particularly noteworthy for their illustrations. Without doubt, the outstanding English textbook of anatomy is that by Henry Gray (1827-1861), which was available in both English and American editions for well over one hundred years, and is still the standard textbook in England, the current thirty-eighth edition having been published in 1980. Gray was lecturer in anatomy at St. George's Hospital, but died of smallpox at the early age of thirty-four, just after the publication of the second edition of *Anatomy, descriptive and surgical*, which was first published in London in 1858. The book was illustrated by Henry Vandyke Carter (1831-1897) (Plate 48) who later made several important contributions to medical literature when working in India. The second edition contained several new drawings by John Guise Westmacott (1811-1884), but the book has been particularly valued for the engravings from Carter's drawings, many of which survived in successive editions up to 1966.

Medical photography must be treated as an entirely different subject, but it is obvious that photography has been used extensively in medical book illustration. The reproduction of woodcuts and engravings, for example, in reprints and later editions, was frequently achieved by photographic means, the resultant prints being half-tone reproductions, and lithography was similarly employed. Actual photographs were occasionally employed in book illustration, but they did not prove satisfactory either commercially or technically, especially in the early stages, and later developments proved that photographs can be "faked", re-touched, high-lighted, distorted, superimposed etc., as can drawings, to give results that were "unscientific", to say the least. Obviously, photographic reproduction has limitations which can be obviated by the employment of medical artists, but the camera has advantages in more recently-developed techniques applied to scientific purposes. The production of moving pictures, of instant prints, and the application of photography to the microscope, and in electronmicroscopy, immediately come to mind. These and other photographic techniques can assist medical artists in the preparation of drawings which can then be executed more leisurely, and can be adapted to the specific needs of the scientist or customer.

Many of these innovations were introduced in the twentieth century, which was to see many changes in the field of medical book illustration, some being improvements, while others, mainly concerned with medical publication and book production, can be regarded only as retrograde steps.

⇒⊰ CHAPTER 8 ⊱⇐

THE TWENTIETH CENTURY

"The accomplished medical artist ... should be able to compete with the camera on its own terms. He must know how to depict both normal and abnormal tissues with the greatest of realism. He must be able to impart just the right sheen to a picture of the cranial dura, or proper dullness to an infected area of the peritoneum. He should have the skill to make the whole picture look solid and real and three dimensional, to make one structure stand out in front of another."

Frank H. Netter.

No epoch-making invention or variation in technique was introduced to provide a sharp demarcation between nineteenth-century and twentieth-century medical book illustration, and one century slid gently into the next. Neither medical artists nor medical photographers achieved professional recognition until the twentieth century was well advanced, but the need for their services, at least on a part-time or free-lance basis, had long been established. In 1842 W. A. Delamotte was employed at St. Bartholomew's Hospital to instruct students in anatomical drawing, using the Reading Room for his classes. He was later appointed as the first Librarian, combining his duties with that of Artist, until he was replaced by Thomas Godart in 1852. In 1881 Godart asked for the offices of Librarian and Artist to be separated, and he continued to make his drawings in the Curator's Room. A "photographic apparatus" was purchased in 1882, and Godart was also appointed as photographer, but he finally retired in 1887 and went to Australia, where he died shortly after his arrival. He illustrated Luther Holden's *Human osteology* and many other books.

Similar schemes probably operated in other medical schools, with drawings made by anybody capable of wielding a brush or pen, including many medical men, some of whom were very talented artists. Photographs were provided in a similar manner, and, even in the twentieth century, secretaries also provided drawings and wielded the camera. Photographers and artists depicting medical subjects were initially introduced through their employment by individual medical men for specific tasks, such as the illustration of books and articles. Later they were attached to departments to provide teaching material for museums, exhibitions, lectures and wall-charts. Where several departments were similarly interested, it became obvious that a separate department would prove more economical, but this was a later development, and has obviously presented many problems which are inevitable in the sharing of services, finance and staff.

A synopsis of the use made by Sir James Purves-Stewart (1869-1949) of the application of photography to medicine has been written by Peter Hansell

(1977). Some of Purves-Stewart's photographs were featured in the first edition of his *Diagnosis of nervous diseases*, published in 1906, which went into many editions and translations. Almost 200 clinical photographs illustrate the book, some of which show evidence of blocking-out, air-brushing and other graphic techniques. Purves-Stewart was among the inventive pioneers of medical photography, and later used cinematography in his neurological investigations. During World War I he used soldiers as his clinical material, and in 1946 he became a founder member of the Medical Group of the Royal Photographic Society.

The reproduction of X-ray photographs presented many problems at the turn of the century. Half-tone blocks of radiographs often proved unsatisfactory because of the prohibitive cost of making prints large enough to show sufficient detail, and to print them on the good-quality paper necessary to achieve successful results. Sylvia Treadgold (1954) suggested that many of these could be better expressed by drawings suitable for reproduction as line-blocks. These are made either by tracing original radiographs, or by inking in the outline on a contact print and then bleaching out the photographic image. Both black and white embossed scraper-board can be used, but the former should not be reproduced as half-tone blocks, and black greasy chalk should be used on the white scraper-board. Sylvia Treadgold (1954) provides examples of these techniques in illustrations by Pamela Carter.

Although the introduction of photography and subsequent improvements in techniques suggested that this medium would replace the artist, on the grounds that the camera "never lies", or misleads the viewer, films and plates can be "re-touched", and "trick" photography can produce the "effects" required by the manipulator. This nullifies the suggestion that the photograph is more "scientific" and shows every detail as it occurs naturally. Even with elaborate lighting, it is difficult for the camera, without special equipment, to penetrate the inner recesses exposed in surgical operations, and it obviously cannot ignore unimportant detail and highlight the sections of particular interest to the surgeon. However, the camera can assist the artist, and the artist can improve photographs and aid the photographer in many other ways.

The most important figure in the development of medical illustration in the twentieth century was undoubtedly Max Brödel (1870-1941). As a student in Leipzig he had studied the basic principles of art work, and particularly lithography, and his first medical drawing was made for Carl Friedrich Wilhelm Ludwig (1816-1895). Brödel also made anatomical drawings for Christian Wilhelm Braune (1831-1892) and Karl Werner Spalteholz (1861-1940), and while still in Leipzig he first heard of the Johns Hopkins Medical School in Baltimore. He went there in 1894 to concentrate on medical illustration, to be joined by his friend Herman Becker, and a few years later, by another friend, August Horn. These three worked together as a team, and in 1911 Brödel founded the Art Department at Johns Hopkins. This attracted many pupils, including members of the medical profession, medical students, and also artists. Max Brödel (1941) wrote an interesting article outlining his own career, describing the establishment of the Art Department, and providing information on the training of medical artists. He worked for Howard A. Kelly, illustrating several books and articles by him, and also with Thomas S. Cullen, and others. Rainer M. Engel (1969) has contributed an appreciation of Brödel's contribution to medical illustration, and five of his drawings, with those of some of his pupils, were reproduced in a report on an art exhibition (Brödel, 1956). Another American medical artist of distinction, Thomas S. Jones, has written an interesting article on the history of the subject (Jones, 1959) in which he brought the subject up to date by mentioning the other artists of this century, including Henry Faber and his two sons Ludwig and Erwin, who illustrated many medical books, including George Arthur Piersol's *Human anatomy*, first published in 1907.

The first student at the Art Department from England was Audrey J. Arnott, who was sent from Oxford with an introductory letter from (Sir) Hugh Cairns (1896-1952), who had studied with Harvey Cushing in Boston, and she spent six months there. Max Brödel adapted Ross Board, a chalk surface paper, for medical drawing, and Audrey Arnott taught the technique to Margaret C. McLarty, who also worked in Oxford. They illustrated a series of books for the Nuffield Department of Anaesthetics, and made many drawings for illustrations in books by Sir Robert Macintosh, Hamilton Bailey, Rodney Maingot and others. Margaret MacLarty (1960) in her book *Illustrating medicine and surgery*, has provided information on the early history of the subject, with significant sections on training, equipment, techniques and other aspects of the work of the medical artist.

Before World War II there was little literature on the subject of medical illustration, but following that event there was a renewed interest in the work of medical artists and photographers. Carl P. Rollins (1949), in an article on illustration in printed medical books, surveyed the historical scene, following this with a summary of the impact of lithographic processes such as chromolithography, coloured aquatint, photoengravings in line, which were first introduced in 1877, and were similar to wood-blocks, and a few years later were followed by half-tones. Half-tones were produced by the use of two glass plates, on the surfaces of which were etched parallel lines (400 lines or fewer to the inch), the two plates then being placed so that the lines crossed at right angles. This resulted in a multitude of small, irregular dots when the print was filtered through the screen. Other photographic processes include photogravure, a photo-mechanical engraving process; rotogravure, in which a copper-plate is attached to a web of paper; heliotype or collotype, which is produced by photographing the image on a sensitized piece of plate glass, and printing by a lithographic process. The use of colour filters was introduced in 1890, and resulted in four separate negatives and printing plates, yellow, red, blue and black, the last being printed to intensify the whole. In the offset process the picture is transferred to a sheet of zinc, and the printing is first done on a rubber-covered cylinder, from which it is transferred to paper.

Sylvia Treadgold (1949) has outlined the work of the medical illustrator, indicating the wide potential in the production of displays, exhibitions, graphs, wall charts, pamphlets for patients, posters, etc., in addition to the activities normally associated with a medical artist. Her article also describes materials and methods. Robert Ollerenshaw (1955-56) provided a short history of medical illustration in an article which suggested that the "present tendency to force everything into graphs and histograms will also settle down"; and "the division of illustration into art and photography is unreal". The latter quotation was expanded in a later publication by Ollerenshaw (1957):

> "It matters not whether a piece of illustrative material be made with a pencil, a brush, a camera, some wax, or carved on the cliffs of Dover with a pickaxe: the crux of the matter is its fitness for the purpose for which it was commissioned, and there is no place in medical illustration today for Photography or Art spelt with capital letters, each seeking where it can score off the other". (p. 551).

Another historical survey published by Robert Ollerenshaw (1965) as the shortened version of the first Henry Lecture given to the Royal College of Surgeons in Ireland, is illustrated with a small selection of the numerous slides shown at the lecture, and it also suggests the author's views on a currently-popular term:

> "I dislike intensely the term 'visual aids', but if it is to be used then let it be clearly understood that it implies aid to the student and not to his teacher".

Peter Cull (1978) has more recently published a precise summary of the many uses of visual information in medical teaching, illustrating it with examples of actual photography of skin disease in a patient; superficial dissection of the head and thorax as interpreted by an artist; an imaginative progressive dissection of the orbits (Plate 49); a diagrammatic representation of chemical action; and the discreet use of humour to emphasize a salient fact by means of a cartoon. The last is reproduced here (Plate 50) as an excellent example of the employment of caricature in teaching medicine, a technique recently re-introduced in medical literature, particularly in students' textbooks. The use of diagrams, charts, histograms, "manikins" and "matchstick men" are also used to explain the text, and represent a reversion to the simple technique expressed in pictographs. This is partly due to the time required to produce sophisticated, detailed drawings, which have become more rare in medical book illustration with the need for speedy publication. Wall charts for teaching anatomy and other subjects have survived, and are useful for display in dissection rooms, lecture theatres, museums and libraries, and the combination of photography and diagrammatic drawing is illustrated in Plate 51.

The work of the medical book illustrator is greatly influenced by modern methods of book production. William Hunter's *Gravid uterus*, printed in 1774 at the Baskerville Press, with ink and paper specially made for the project, took over twenty years from the preparation of the first drawing to publication in book form. Today, type and illustrations can be printed together by a modern press such as a Harris M200A five unit, twin web, heat-set press which can print

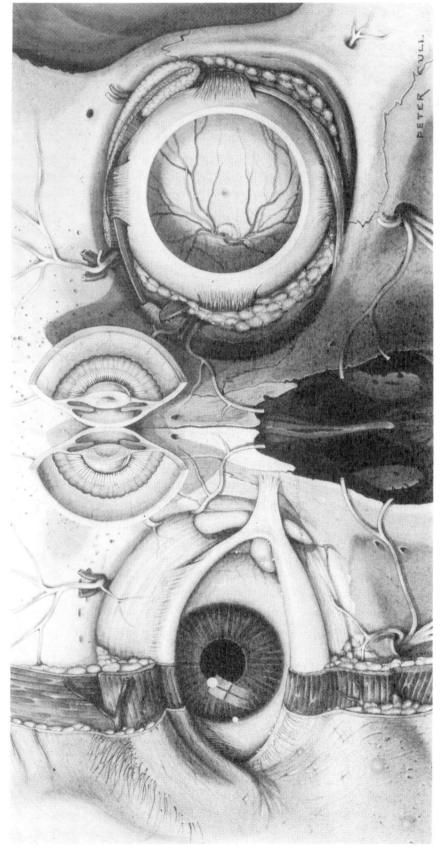

Plate 49. Drawing by Peter Cull showing a progressive dissection of the orbits. (By permission of the artist).

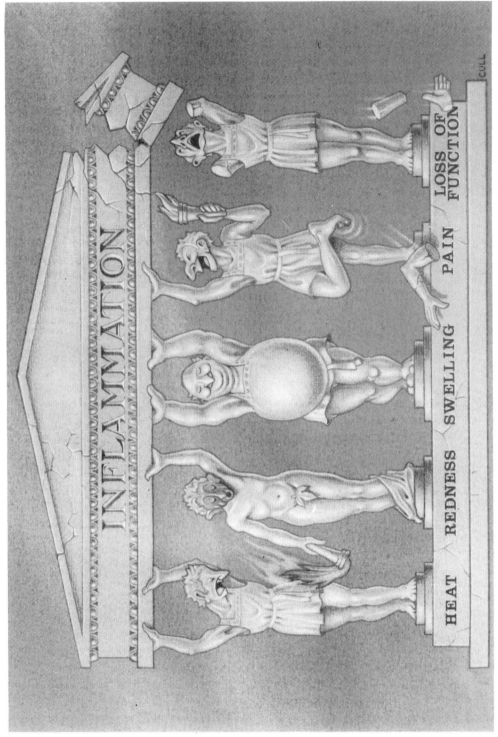

Plate 50. Use of humour in medical education. The cardinal sins of inflammation, by Peter Cull. (By permission of the artist).

one web in four colours both sides and black on the other web, or two colours on both sides of each web in one pass through the machine. Typesetting is keyboarded to produce a punched paper tape, which operates the computer unit. Colour separation is by electronic scanning, and ink strength is controlled by a 'Telecolour' colour console. The technical equipment is complicated and expensive, and the resultant book, although of improved technical quality, is usually not published more cheaply or more quickly than by the older orthodox methods. The process is employed to advantage in the printing of journals, particularly those carrying extensive advertising material. It is a curious fact that, for many years, colour illustrations in advertisements in medical journals have been far better produced than those in the text, and those in medical books. One reason was the fact that the advertisements were printed on better paper. Also, many medical books had to be printed abroad, not only for better quality of printing, but for comparative cheapness.

German anatomical atlases have been outstanding for their illustrations for many years. Urban & Schwarzenberg (1977) held an exhibition showing the history of medical illustration over the previous eighty years. The published catalogue is profusely illustrated with anatomical and histological drawings, as well as wood engravings, and describes the various methods of reproduction, indicating their development over the years. It gives details of some of the artists, providing examples of their work, and comparing the treatment of similar subjects by various artists.

Erich Lepier (1900-1974) first painted miniatures, and was largely self-taught. In 1924 he joined Urban & Schwarzenberg, and as a freelance he made drawings for several medical men, including Eduard Pernkopf. During the next twenty years he made many of the drawings for Pernkopf's *Topographische Anatomie des Menschen*, four volumes, 1937-1960 (Plate 52). Several other artists were involved in this project, including Karl Endtresser, and Franz Batke (born 1903), who also made 371 drawings for *Die vaginalen Operationen* by Günther Reiffenstuhl and Werner Platzer, published in 1974. Carl Toldt's *Anatomische Atlas für Studierende und Ärzte*, nine parts, Vienna, 1896-1900, contains wood-engravings, mostly from drawings by Fritz Meixner, many of which still appeared in the twenty-sixth edition. It contains over 1400 illustrations, for which the drawings were photographically transferred to wood block, and then engraved. In his *Atlas der descriptiven Anatomie des Menschen*, two volumes, Vienna and Leipzig, 1902-1905, Carl Heitzmann drew directly on the wood from the specimens, the blocks then being engraved. All the illustrations in the first edition of Johannes Sobotta's *Atlas der descriptiven Anatomie des Menschen*, Munich, 1904-1907, were drawn by Karl Hajek, and many are still included in the latest English edition (1974), which also has illustrations by Erich Lepier.

Wars have always tended to stimulate surgical research, and have also provided employment for war artists, the combination of the two being particularly evident during World Wars I and II. Henry Tonks (1862-1937) later became Slade Professor of Fine Art at University College, London, but he had also qualified as a surgeon, and his talents in both disciplines are

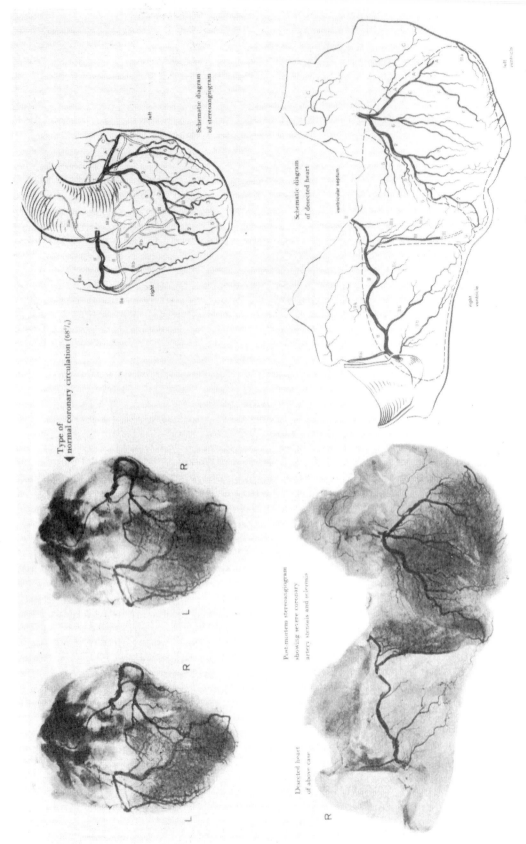

Plate 51. Section of wall chart, "Topography and nomenclature of coronary circulation in arteriograms", showing stereograms and schematic diagrams of the heart. (By permission of Schering).

perpetuated in his pastel drawings made for Sir Harold Delf Gillies (1882-1960) and Sir William Kelsey Fry (1889-1963). Tonks provided some of the illustrations for Gillies' *Plastic surgery of the face*, 1920, four of his original drawings being in the Royal College of Surgeons of England Library, and thirty being deposited with the Royal Army Dental Corps. The Royal College of Surgeons houses many other drawings of medical subjects by Anna Zinkeisen and others.

Frank H. Netter has become the best-known American medical artist of recent years, mainly because of his remarkable illustrations in the *CIBA Collection of Medical Illustrations*. These cover many medical and surgical subjects, and have proved immensely popular (Plate 53). His early life and training both as an artist and surgeon, and his connection with the CIBA Pharmaceutical Company, have been described in a recent article (Netter, 1981). Frank H. Netter (1949) had earlier described his own method of working

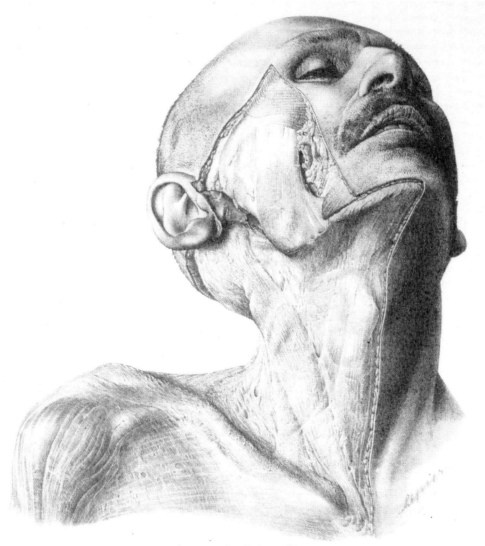

Plate 52. Drawing by Erich Lepier, from Pernkopf's *Topographische Anatomie des Menschen*. *(Urban and Schwarzenberg)*.

121

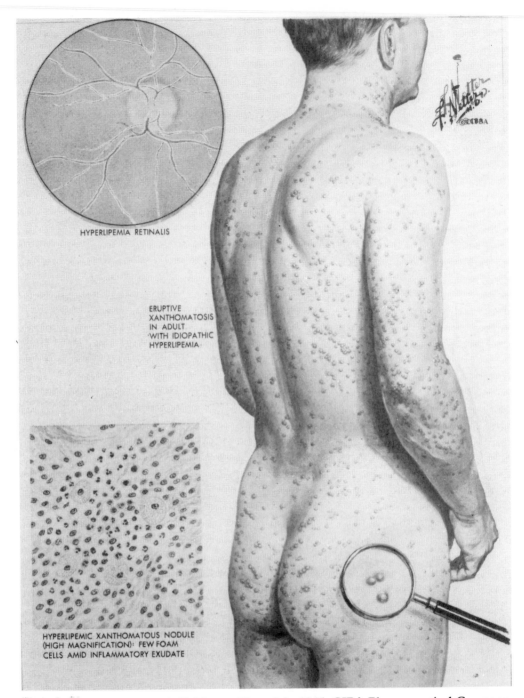

HYPERLIPEMIA RETINALIS

ERUPTIVE
XANTHOMATOSIS
IN ADULT
WITH IDIOPATHIC
HYPERLIPEMIA

HYPERLIPEMIC XANTHOMATOUS NODULE
(HIGH MAGNIFICATION): FEW FOAM
CELLS AMID INFLAMMATORY EXUDATE

Plate 53. Drawing by Frank H. Netter. (Copyright 1965, CIBA Pharmaceutical Company, Division of CIBA-GEIGY Corporation. *Reprinted with permission from The CIBA Collection of Medical Illustrations illustrated by Frank H. Netter, M.D. All rights reserved.*)

as a medical artist, giving illustrations of the various stages, and had also written on the history of medical illustration (Netter, 1956 and 1957). He was responsible for the enormous transparent figure of a woman, seven feet high, at the San Francisco Golden Gate Exposition. The various organs were illuminated, and a synchronised voice described their various functions.

A. Kirkpatrick Maxwell was born in Annan in Scotland in 1884, and became interested in art at an early age. He worked as a lithographer in his grandfather's firm, and later was apprenticed to a lithographer in Glasgow, where he also attended evening classes in art. He also illustrated a book on biology for Dr. Bles of the Department of Zoology in Glasgow University, gaining a reputation as an illustrator which led to his becoming a war artist throughout World War I. He produced over 1,000 drawings of war injuries, which were housed in the Royal College of Surgeons, but were unfortunately destroyed during World War II. He did much freelance work while working part-time in the Department of Anatomy at University College, London, under Sir Grafton Elliot Smith (1871-1937), for whom he was making drawings to illustrate a textbook of anatomy which was never completed. Maxwell again served as a war artist during World War II, but then moved to Cambridge, where he illustrated successive editions of *Human embryology* by W. J. Hamilton, J. D. Boyd and H. W. Mossman. Maxwell produced drawings for many other books and articles, including modern editions of Gray's *Anatomy*, and he must be regarded as the outstanding British medical artist of modern times (Plate 54). An account of his life and work, with examples of his drawings, has been published by R. M. S. Bell and A. E. Clark-Kennedy (1973). Maxwell used white paint to produce highlights, and also used the airbrush, a technique patented in Britain by Charles L. Burdick. The use of this was revived in the 1960s, when Peter Cull was one of the first artists to use it in medical illustration: another was Douglas Kidd in Liverpool.

Anna Zinkeisen worked as an official war artist during World War II, and while at St. Mary's Hospital, Paddington, started a course in medical illustration at St. Martin's School of Art. Some of her drawings are preserved in the Royal College of Surgeons of England Library, and others were reproduced in *Anna: a memorial tribute to Anna Zinkeisen*, by Josephine Walpole, published in a limited edition by Royle Publications in 1978. Clifford Shepley started a short-lived school of medical illustration at Edinburgh University, and wrote an excellent article on the development of the subject (Shepley, 1951). These are but a few of the medical artists who have been, and still are, providing illustrations in medical publications. They are scattered throughout the medical centres, and particularly in medical schools where medical illustration and audio-visual departments have been created; they have contributed effectively to the improvement of medical illustrations in all forms; and they have also trained others to follow in their footsteps.

Although widely dispersed, medical illustrators have been linked together by membership of various organizations formed for this purpose. In the United States of America, the Association of Medical Illustrators (A.M.I.) was established in 1945 to further the study of medical illustration, and to encourage the development of visual aids in medical education. It holds an annual meeting, and every third year joins with the Biological Photographic Association and the Health Sciences Communications Association (H.S.C.A.) for a joint convention. The A.M.I. and the H.S.C.A. publish jointly the *Journal of Biocommunication*, and the A.M.I. sets standards for the training of medical illustrators at accredited schools.

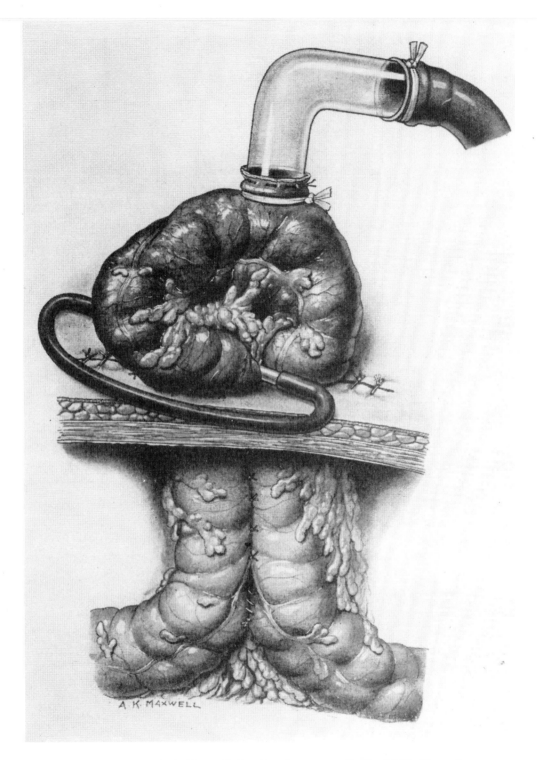

Plate 54. Drawing by A.K. Maxwell showing first stage of a Paul-Mikulicz colostomy.

In Britain, the Medical Artists Association was founded in 1949, and awards a diploma following extensive study and practical experience under supervision, completed by the submission of a suitable thesis. The Institute of Medical and Biological Illustration (I.M.B.I.) originated in 1968 following meetings of six medical photographers and six medical artists. Peter Hansell, Gabriel Donald, Peter Cull and Norman K. Harrison were the first honorary officers in the organization. Training schemes are run by various bodies, and qualifications are awarded by the City and Guilds of London Institute, and the Institute of Incorporated Photographers. The official organ of the I.M.B.I. is *Journal of Audiovisual Media in Medicine*, which was originally *Medical and Biological Illustration*, and the Institute holds an annual conference for its members, which includes those working in agriculture, biology, botany, medicine, veterinary science, and zoology.

Similar organizations exist in other parts of the world, and James Ho (1981) has described the organization of medical illustration services in Japan, Korea, Philippines, Thailand, Vietnam and Hong Kong, many of which are being modernised. He also gives a brief description of early Chinese medicine, and suggests that it may soon be possible to publish a journal devoted to medical illustration in the Far East.

Personal libraries have declined in numbers and in the nature of their contents. "Paperbacks" have largely replaced "cased" books, and finely bound volumes have been relegated to presentations and commemorative items. Good bookbinders capable of binding books in leather are difficult to locate, and the resultant volumes are correspondingly rare. The decline of the apprentice craftsman (in most trades) since the outbreak of World War II has resulted in fewer personnel with a thorough knowledge of their craft, and a greater reliance on technical machinery. Some books appear only in paperback form, but where some of the edition is cased, there is a wide difference in the prices of the two issues which bears no relation to the comparative cost of casing large numbers of books by machine, as opposed to conventional binding. Most libraries, and many individuals, prefer books in hardback, particularly if they are to be retained for long periods, but they are not prepared to pay almost double the price for them.

Beautiful books with attractive illustrations reproduced on good quality paper in hardback are becoming scarce, mainly owing to the high costs of production and marketing, and the inevitable high prices. Fewer individuals purchase books other than the expendable paperbacks, and there is a need for pupils at school, students and others to be taught not only how to use books, but to encourage an appreciation of them as physical objects. Attractively produced, they can give pleasure as well as knowledge, and encourage the development of a personal library of which one can be proud. The ownership of books can also prove a sound investment. They may not become literary classics, but if well-illustrated and attractively produced, they will be in demand long after the original publisher has allowed them to go out of print.

Computerised mechanical aids to book production involve the expenditure of large sums of money, and the financial combines owning most of the larger

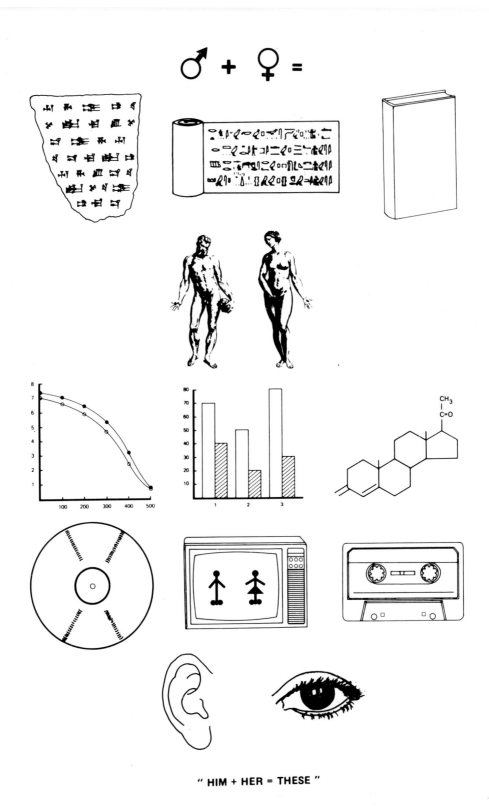

Plate 55. The rise and decline of medical illustration.

printers and publishers expect to make profits quickly for shareholders. The need to recoup capital quickly and make high profits results in high prices, and specialised books which should be available for many years are often quickly remaindered if not sold within a few months of publication. This suggests that there is a need for small publishers and printers to produce books which are bibliographically attractive, enshrining the scholarship of the author, embellished with the work of the artists, and reproduced with materials that have not been manufactured solely for the convenience of mechanical robots.

We have briefly traced the evolution of medical illustration from the primitive scripts and pictographs through the various forms and techniques of book illustration, and highlighted the artists and craftsmen of the period when medical book illustration was at its peak. Recent years have seen the return of the pictograph, the diagrammatic, "matchstick-men", audiovisual aids in the form of tapes and television, drawing by computers, and a decline in the number of books which will be valued mainly for their illustrations (Plate 55). Fortunately, there are more artists capable of portraying medical subjects, and of lending their talents to all forms of medical education requiring artistic interpretation. They will benefit from studying the work of their predecessors, by appreciating the lengthy history of their subject, and by ensuring the continuity of their profession as a major auxiliary to medical education.

✦ BIBLIOGRAPHY ✦

This is a selective list of references used in the preparation of this book, most of which are noted in the text by the name of the author followed by the date of publication in parenthesis. Additional material can be traced by reference to Thornton (1966), Thornton and Tully (1971-78), the Wellcome Institute for the History of Medicine *Subject catalogue of the history of medicine and related sciences*, 17 vols., Munich, *Kraus*, 1980, and to *Current Work in the History of Medicine*.

Aldis, Harry G. (1941). *The printed book. The second edition revised and brought up to date by John Carter and E. A. Crutchley*. Cambridge, *University Press*, 1941.

Anderson, William (1886). An outline of the history of art in its relation to medical science. *St. Thomas's Hospital Reports*, 15, 1886, pp. 151-181.

Audette, Louis G. (1979). Stylism in anatomical illustration from the sixteenth to the twentieth centuries. *Journal of Biocommunication*, 6, 1979, pp. 24-29, 34-37.

Bell, R. M. S., and Clark-Kennedy, A. E. (1973). A. Kirkpatrick Maxwell: an illustrated appreciation. *Medical and Biological Illustration*, 23, 1973, pp. 17-22.

Belt, Elmer (1955). *Leonardo the anatomist*. Lawrence, Kansas, *University of Kansas Press*, 1955. (Logan Clendening Lectures on the History of Medicine. Fourth Series).

Bishop, W. J. (1954). Antonio Scarpa, 1752-1832. *Medical and Biological Illustration*, 4, 1954, pp. 7-9.

Blunt, Wilfrid (1950). *The art of botanical illustration. By Wilfrid Blunt, with the assistance of William T. Stearn*. London, *Collins*, 1950.

Breasted, James Henry (1950). *A history of Egypt*. London, New York, *Scribner*, 1950.

Brödel, Max (1941). Medical illustration. *Journal of the American Medical Association*, 117, 1941, pp. 668-672.

Brödel, Max (1956). [Examples of medical illustration by Max Brödel and some of his students.] *Postgraduate Medicine*, 19, 1956, pp. 86-89.

Carter, Thomas Francis (1955). *The invention of printing in China and its spread westward. . . . Revised by L. Carrington Goodrich. Second edition.* New York, *Ronald*, 1955.

Castiglione, Arturo (1958). *A history of medicine.* New York, *Knopf*, 1958.

Chen, Chan-Yuen (1969). *History of Chinese medical science: illustrated with pictures.* Hong Kong, *Chinese Medical Institute*, 1969.

Choulant, Ludwig (1945). *History and bibliography of anatomic illustration . . . Translated and annotated by Mortimer Frank. Further essays by Fielding H. Garrison, Mortimer Frank, Edward C. Streeter, with a new historical essay by Charles Singer, and a bibliography of Mortimer Frank by J. Christian Bay.* New York, London, *Hafner*, 1945, (reprinted 1962). (First German edition, 1852).

Coleman, Ruth B. (1950). Illustration of human anatomy before Vesalius. *Surgery, Gynecology and Obstetrics*, 9, 1950, pp. 500-507.

Cope, *Sir* Zachary (1953). *William Cheselden, 1688-1752.* Edinburgh, *Livingstone*, 1953.

Crummer, LeRoy (1926). The copper plates in Raynalde and Geminus. *Proceedings of the Royal Society of Medicine*, 20, 1926, Sect. Hist. Med., pp. 53-56.

Cule, John (1980). *A doctor for the people: 2000 years of general practice in Britain.* London, [etc.], *Update Books*, 1980.

Cull, Peter (1978). Illustration in medical teaching. *Journal of Audiovisual Media in Medicine*, 1, 1978 pp. 180-181.

Cushing, Harvey (1962). *A bio-bibliography of Andreas Vesalius . . . Second edition.* Hamden, Conn., London, *Archon Books*, 1962.

De Lint, J. G. (1916). The plates of Jenty. *Janus*, 21, 1916, pp. 129-135.

Dobson, Jessie (1954). *William Clift.* London, *Heinemann*, 1954.

Doherty, Terence (1974). *The anatomical works of George Stubbs.* London, *Secker & Warburg*, 1974.

Duff, E. Gordon (1893). *Early printed books.* London, *Kegan Paul, Trench, Trübner*, 1893. (Books about Books Series).

Engel, Rainer M. (1969). Max Brödel (1870-1941). *Investigative Urology*, 7, 1969, pp. 192-193.

Fountain, R. B. (1968). George Stubbs (1724-1806) as an anatomist. *Proceedings of the Royal Society of Medicine*, 61, 1968, pp. 639-646.

Gaunt, William (1977). *Stubbs.* London, *Phaidon*, 1977.

Gibson, William Carleton (1970). The bio-medical pursuits of Christopher Wren. *Medical History*, 14, 1970, pp. 331-341.

Goldscheider, Ludwig (1959). *Leonardo da Vinci: life and work, paintings and drawings. With the Leonardo biography by Vasari, 1568. (Sixth edition).* London, *Phaidon Press*, 1959. (First edition, 1943).

Gordon-Taylor, *Sir* Gordon, and Walls, E. W. (1958). *Sir Charles Bell, his life and times.* Edinburgh, London, *Livingstone,* 1958.

Greim, Florence M. (1952). Anatomical illustrations from the Fothergill Collections at the Pennsylvania Hospital, with a foreword by Florence M. Greim. *What's New,* April, 1952.

Guerra, Francisco (1969). The identity of the artists involved in Vesalius's *Fabrica,* 1543. *Medical History,* 13, 1969, pp. 37-50.

Hahn, André, *et al.* (1962). *Histoire de la médecine et du livre médical, à la lumière des collections de la Bibliothèque de la Faculté de Paris. André Hahn, Paule Dumaître, avec la collaboration de Janine Samion-Contet.* Paris, *Olivier Perrin,* 1962.

Hansell, Peter (1977). A backward glance. *Medical and Biological Illustration,* 27, 1977, pp. 137-139.

Harthan, John (1981). *The history of the illustrated book. The western tradition.* London, *Thames and Hudson,* 1981.

Herrlinger, Robert (1970). *History of medical illustration from antiquity to A.D. 1600.* London, *Pitman,* 1970.

Hill, T. G. (1915). *The essentials of illustration. A practical guide to the reproduction of drawings & photographs for the use of scientists & others.* London, *Wesley,* 1915.

Ho, James (1981). Medical illustration in the Far East. *Journal of Audiovisual Media in Medicine,* 4, 1981, pp. 58-61.

Huard, Pierre, and Wong, Ming (1959). *La Médecine chinoise au cours des siècles.* Paris, *Roger Dacosta,* 1959. (English translation, 1968).

Hurry, Jamieson B. (1928). *Imhotep. Second edition.* Oxford, *University Press,* 1928.

Hutchison, Harold F. (1975) *Sir Christopher Wren: a biography.* London, *Gollancz,* 1975.

Jones, Harold Wellington (1937). Charles Bell and the origin of his engravings of the arteries. *Medical Life,* 44, 1937, pp. 372-380.

Jones, Thomas S. (1959). The story of medical illustration. *Journal of the International College of Surgeons,* 32, 1959, pp. 697-707.

Kan, Lai-Bing (1965). Introduction to Chinese medical literature, *Bulletin of the Medical Library Association,* 53, 1965, pp. 60-70.

Keynes, *Sir* Geoffrey L. (1953). *A bibliography of the writings of Dr. William Harvey, 1578-1657. . . . Second edition, revised.* Cambridge, *University Press,* 1953.

Keynes, *Sir* Geoffrey L. (1966). *The life of William Harvey.* Oxford, *Clarendon Press,* 1966.

Keys, Thomas E. (1940). The earliest medical books printed with movable type: a review. *Library Quarterly,* 10, 1940, pp. 220-230.

Knox, Robert (1852). *Great artists and great anatomists; a biographical and philosophical study.* London, *John Van Voorst*, 1852.

Krivatsy, Peter (1968). Le Blon's anatomical colour engravings. *Journal of the History of Medicine*, 23, 1968, pp. 153-158.

Krumbhaar, Edward B. (1922). The early history of anatomy in the United States. *Annals of Medical History*, 4, 1922, pp. 271-286.

Lambert, Samuel W., Wiegand, Willy, and Ivins, William M. (1952). *Three Vesalian essays to accompany the Icones Anatomicae of 1934.* New York, *Macmillan*, 1952.

LeFanu, William R. (1952). *A bio-bibliography of Edward Jenner, 1749-1823.* London, *Harvey and Blythe*, 1951.

LeFanu, William R. (1960). Anatomical drawings by Jacobus Schijnvoet. *Oud Holland*, 1960, pp. 54-58.

LeFanu, William R. (1961). Charles Bell and Cheselden. *Medical History*, 5, 1961, p. 165.

LeFanu, William R. (1971). William Clift. *Dictionary of Scientific Biography*, 3, 1971, pp. 323-325.

LeFanu, William R. (1972). Some English illustrated medical books. *Book Collector*, 21, 1972, pp. 19-28.

LeFanu, William R. (1976). *Notable medical books from the Lilly Library, Indiana University.* Indianapolis, *Lilly Research Laboratories*, 1976.

Loechel, William E. (1960). The history of medical illustration. *Bulletin of the Medical Library Association*, 48, 1960, pp. 168-171.

Lumsden, E. S. (1962). *The art of etching. A complete & fully illustrated description of etching, drypoint, soft-ground etching, aquatint & their allied arts, together with technical notes upon their own work by many of the leading etchers of the present time.* New York, *Dover Publications*, 1962. (First published in 1924).

MacKinney, Loren C. (1949). Medical illustration, ancient and medieval. *CIBA Symposium*, 10, 1949, pp. 1062-1071.

MacKinney, Loren C. (1965). *Medical illustrations in medieval manuscripts, Part I. Early medicine in illustrated manuscripts. Part II. Medical miniatures in extant manuscripts: a checklist compiled with the assistance of Thomas Herndon.* London, *Wellcome Historical Medical Library*, 1965.

McLarty, Margaret C. (1960). *Illustrating medicine and surgery.* Edinburgh, London, *Livingstone*, 1960.

Madan, Falconer (1893). *Books in manuscript: a short introduction to their study and use. With a chapter on records.* London, *Kegan Paul, Trench and Trübner*, 1893. (Books about Books Series).

Margotta, Roberto (1968). *A history of medicine.* London, *Paul Hamlyn*, 1968.

Mertz, Barbara (1964). *Temples, tombs and hieroglyphs.* London, *Victor Gollancz*, 1964.

Nasr, Seyyed Hossein (1976). *Islamic science: an illustrated study*. London, *World of Islam Festival Publishing Company*, 1976.

Nathan, Helmuth M. (1976). Art in medicine. *New York State Journal of Medicine*, 76, 1976, pp. 1135-1140.

Netter, Frank H. (1949). A medical illustrator at work. *CIBA Symposium*, 10, 1949, pp. 1087-1092.

Netter, Frank H. (1956). Medical illustration: its history and present day practice. *Journal of the International College of Surgeons*, 26, 1956, pp. 505-513.

Netter, Frank H. (1957). Medical illustration: its history, significance and practice. *Bulletin of the New York Academy of Medicine*, 33, 1957, pp. 357-368.

Netter, Frank H. (1981). Frank Netter: the man, the artist, the surgeon. *Medical Times*, 109, 1981, pp. 31-33.

Ober, William B. (1970). George Stubbs, 1724-1806: mirror up to nature. *New York State Journal of Medicine*, 70, 1970, pp. 986-992.

Ollerenshaw, Robert (1952). The decorated woodcut initials of Vesalius' "Fabrica". *Medical and Biological Illustration*, 2, 1952, pp. 160-166.

Ollerenshaw, Robert (1955-56). Medical illustration. *Transactions of the Medical Society of London*, 72, 1955-56, pp. 219-226.

Ollerenshaw, Robert (1957). Medical illustration: prospect and retrospect. *British Journal of Photography*, 104, 1957, pp. 550-551.

Ollerenshaw, Robert (1965). Better than a thousand words: a survey of medical illustration today. The first Henry Lecture to the Royal College of Surgeons in Ireland. *Journal of the Royal College of Surgeons in Ireland*, 1, 1965, pp. 171-185.

Ollerenshaw, Robert (1974). Dr. Hunter's 'Gravid uterus' — a bicentenary note. *Medical and Biological Illustration*, 24, 1974, pp. 43-57.

Ollerenshaw, Robert (1977). The camera obscura in medical illustration: a belated reference. *British Journal of Photography*, 1977, pp. 815-816.

O'Malley, Charles D. (1964). *Andreas Vesalius of Brussels, 1514-1564*. Berkeley, Los Angeles, *University of California Press*, 1964.

O'Malley, Charles D., and Saunders, J. B. de C. M. (1952). *Leonardo da Vinci on the human body. The anatomical, physiological and embryological drawings of Leonardo da Vinci. With translations, emendations and a biographical introduction by Charles D. O'Malley and J. B. de C. M. Saunders*. New York, *Schuman*, 1952.

Ōtori, Ranzaburō (1964). The acceptance of Western medicine in Japan. *In*, Centre for East Asian Cultural Studies, Tokyo. *Acceptance of Western cultures in Japan from the sixteenth to the mid-nineteenth century*. Tokyo, *Centre for East Asian Cultural Studies*, 1964, pp. 20-40.

Pegus, Lindsey (1978). Leonardo da Vinci — anatomical drawings. *Journal of Audiovisual Media in Medicine*, 1, 1978, pp. 63-69.

Pizon, Pierre (1950). L'Oeuvre anatomique du graveur J. -F. Gautier. *La Presse Médicale*, 58, 1950, pp. 1486-1488.

Pollak, Kurt, and Underwood, E. Ashworth (1968). *The healers: the doctor then and now.* London, *Thomas Nelson*, 1968.

Pollard, Alfred W. (1893). *Early illustrated books: a history of the decoration and illustration of books in the 15th and 16th centuries.* London, *Kegan Paul, Trench, Trübner*, 1893. (Books about Books Series).

Premuda, Loris (1956). *Storia dell' iconografia anatomica.* Milan, *Aldo Martello*, [1956].

Putscher, Marielene (1972). *Geschichte der medizinischen Abbildung. Von 1600 bis zur Gegenwart.* Munich, *Heinz Moos*, 1972. (This follows on from the original German version of Herrlinger (1970), but has not been translated into English.)

Rechung Rinpoche (1973). *Tibetan medicine illustrated in original texts, presented and translated by the Ven. Rechung Rinpoche Jampal Kunzgang.* London, *Wellcome Institute of the History of Medicine*, 1973.

Reeves, Carole (1980). Illustrations of medicine in ancient Egypt. *Journal of Audiovisual Media in Medicine*, 3, 1980, pp. 4-13.

Roberts, K. B. (1981). Maps of the body: anatomical illustration through five centuries. *Memorial University of Newfoundland. Occasional Papers in the History of Medicine*, No. 2, 1981.

Rollins, Carl Purington (1949). Illustration in printed medical books. *CIBA Symposiuim*, 10, 1949, pp. 1072-1086.

Russell, K. F. (1954). The Osteographia of William Cheselden. *Bulletin of the History of Medicine*, 28, 1954, pp. 32-49.

Salvadori, B. A. (1981). Fetal medicine. *Journal of Foetal Medicine*, 1, 1981, pp.1-22.

Saunders, J. B. de C. M., and O'Malley, Charles D. (1973). *The illustrations from the works of Andreas Vesalius of Brussels. With annotations and translations, a discussion of the plates and their background, authorship and influence, and a biographical sketch of Vesalius.* New York, *Dover Publications*, 1973.

Scott, J. A. (1904). Concerning the Fothergill pictures at the Pennsylvania Hospital. *University of Pennsylvania Medical Bulletin*, 16, 1904, pp. 388-393.

Shepley, Clifford (1951). The development of medical illustration. *British Journey of Urology*, 23, 1951, pp. 70-78.

Sigerist, Henry E. (1951-61). *A history of medicine.* Vols. 1 and 2. New York, *Oxford University Press*, 1951-1961.

Singer, Charles, and Underwood, E. Ashworth (1962). *A short history of medicine. Second edition.* Oxford, *Clarendon Press*, 1962.

Slythe, R. Margaret (1970). *The art of illustration, 1750-1900.* London, *Library Association*, 1970.

Swain, Paul (1966). De fistula in ano, by John Arderne (1370): the qualities required in a good surgeon, translated from the Middle-English by Paul Swain. *St. Bartholomew's Hospital Journal*, 70, 1966, pp. 312-317.

Thomas, K. Bryn (1974). The great anatomical atlases. *Proceedings of the Royal Society of Medicine*, 67, 1974, pp. 223-232.

Thompson, Reginald Campbell (1923). *Assyrian medical texts. From the originals in the British Museum.* London, *Oxford University Press*, 1923.

Thompson, Reginald Campbell (1924-26). Assyrian medical texts. *Proceedings of the Royal Society of Medicine*, 17, 1924, Section Hist. Med., pp. 1-34; Part II, 19, 1926, Section Hist. Med., pp. 29-78. (Translations of the facsimiles of medical tablets in Thompson, 1923).

Thornton, John L. (1966). *Medical books, libraries and collectors. A study of bibliography and the book trade in relation to the medical sciences. . . . Second, revised edition.* London, *Deutsch*, 1966.(See also Thornton and Tully, 1971-78).

Thornton, John L. (1982). *Jan Van Rymsdyk, medical artist of the eighteenth century.* Cambridge, New York, *Oleander Press*, 1982.

Thornton, John L., and Tully, R. I. J. (1971-78). *Scientific books, libraries and collectors: a study of bibliography and the book trade in relation to science. Third, revised edition.* London, *Library Association*, 1971 (reprinted 1975). *Supplement 1969-1975*, London, *Library Association*, 1978. (This and Thornton, 1966 contain additional material and references to literature on authors mentioned in the text.)

Thornton, John L., and Want, Patricia C. (1974a). Artist versus engraver in William Hunter's "Anatomy of the human gravid uterus", 1774. *Medical and Biological Illustration*, 24, 1974, pp. 137-139.

Thornton, John L., and Want, Patricia C. (1974b). William Hunter's "The anatomy of the human gravid uterus", 1774-1974. *Journal of Obstetrics and Gynaecology of the British Commonwealth*, 81, 1974, pp. 1-10.

Thornton, John L., and Want, Patricia C. (1978). Charles Nicholas Jenty and the mezzotint plates in his "Demonstrations of a pregnant uterus", 1757. *Journal of Audiovisual Media in Medicine*, 1, 1978, pp. 113-115.

Thornton, John L., and Want, Patricia C. (1979). Jan Van Rymsdyk's illustrations of the gravid uterus drawn for Hunter, Smellie, Jenty and Denman. *Journal of Audiovisual Media in Medicine*, 2, 1979, pp. 10-15.

Thorwald, Jürgen (1962). *Science and secrets of early medicine. Egypt, Mesopotamia, India, China, Mexico.* London, *Thames & Hudson*, 1962.

Treadgold, Sylvia (1949). The scope of the medical illustrator. *Lancet*, 1949 I, pp. 701-704.

Treadgold, Sylvia (1954). Line block reproduction of radiographs. *Medical and Biological Illustration*, 4, 1954, pp. 10-11.

Tsien, Tsuen-Hsuin (1962). *Written on bamboo and silk. The beginnings of Chinese books and inscriptions.* Chicago, *University of Chicago Press*, 1962.

Urban & Schwarzenberg (1977). *The Urban & Schwarzenberg Collection of Medical Illustrations since 1896.* Baltimore, Munich, *Urban & Schwarzenberg*, 1977.

Weindler, Fritz (1908). *Geschichte der gynäkologisch-anatomischen Abbildungen.* Dresden, *Zahn & Jaensch*, 1908.

Wells, Ellen B. (1970). Medical illustration and book decoration in the 18th century. *Medical and Biological Illustration*, 20, 1970, pp. 78-84.

Wells, Ellen B. (1976). Graphic techniques of medical illustration in the 18th century. *Journal of Biocommunication*, 3, 1976, pp. 24-27.

Whillis, J. (1951). Anatomical illustrations. *Medical and Biological Illustration*, 5, 1951, pp. 66-73.

Whitteridge, Gweneth (1971). *William Harvey and the circulation of the blood.* London, *Macdonald*; New York, *American Elsevier*, 1971.

⟡ INDEX ⟡

THE OLEANDER PRESS

JAN VAN RYMSDYK
John L. Thornton
The first biography of the greatest medical artist of the eighteenth century, with twenty plates of his rare and beautiful illustrations to anatomical and gynaecological classics.

A LIFETIME'S READING
Philip Ward
A suggested scheme of reading the world's classics over a fifty-year period, with recommendations on editions and translations, and ideas for musical and artistic appreciation on related themes.

COASTAL FEATURES OF ENGLAND AND WALES
J.A. Steers
Eight new illustrated essays by the author of the standard *Coastline of England and Wales* (C.U.P.), with special reference to cliffs and islands, Thames and Severn, Lancashire, Essex and the Wash.

CELTIC: A COMPARATIVE STUDY
D.B. Gregor
The first detailed comparison of Breton, Cornish, Irish Manx, Scots Gaelic and Welsh, with historical commentary, maps, and photographs. For the general reader as well as the specialist.

ROMONTSCH: LANGUAGE AND LITERATURE
D.B. Gregor
After *Romagnol* and *Friulan*, Douglas Gregor turns his attention to another Romance language: the fourth national language of Switzerland, with a grammar, history, texts and translations.

CAMBRIDGE MUSIC
Frida Knight
The illustrious story of music in Cambridge town, university and county is told here for the first time, with copious illustrations — from Orlando Gibbons to Sir David Willocks.

CAMBRIDGE NEWSPAPERS AND OPINION, 1780-1850
M.J. Murphy
The impact on daily life of the city's early newspapers, shedding fresh light on national politics and society, with plentiful illustrations and a detailed bibliography.

CAMBRIDGE STREET LITERATURE
Philip Ward
The printed ephemera of Cambridge's town and gown are depicted in word and picture by the founder of the Private Libraries Association. The story of almanacks, ballads, playbills and posters.

PETERBOROUGH: A HISTORY
H.F. Tebbs
"The standard reference work" (Peterborough Standard) on the cathedral city and market town which attained new prominence when railways linked it with North and South in the 19th century.

GREGUERIAS
Ramón Gómez de la Serna
The wit and wisdom of the writer claimed by Julián Marias to be the equivalent in modern Spanish literature to Ortega in philosophy, and to Picasso in art. Translations by Philip Ward, author of *The Oxford Companion to Spanish Literature*.

THE OLEANDER PRESS

A DICTIONARY OF COMMON FALLACIES
Philip Ward
Medical, mathematical, biological, astronomical and other fallacies drawn from all fields of human knowledge. "One of the most entertaining reference books ever written" (Daily Telegraph).

THE LIFE AND MURDER OF HENRY MORSHEAD
Ian Morshead
The mystery of the killing of the Everest climber and Survey of India cartographer Morshead has at last been solved, after fifty years, by Morshead's own son. Published by The Oleander Press Ltd.

THE GOLD-MINES OF MIDIAN
Sir Richard Burton
The great explorer's chronicle of a gold search in Arabia is here published, for the first time as the author intended, in the edition by Philip Ward.

KING HUSAIN AND THE KINGDOM OF HEJAZ
Randall Baker
A history of the dynasty which ruled the state now forming the western region of Saudi Arabia, and which also ruled some time in Iraq and Jordan.

TRAVELS IN ARABIA, 1845 and 1848
Yrjö Aukusti Wallin
Pioneering exploration in northern Arabia by a Fenno-Swede writing in English. With new introductory material by W.R. Mead and M. Trautz.

HEJAZ BEFORE WORLD WAR I
D.G. Hogarth
A reprint of the enlarged Arab Bureau of Cairo *Handbook to Hejaz* (1917), with a new introduction by R.L. Bidwell. Even now the best route guide to isolated oases.

ARABIA IN EARLY MAPS
G.R. Tibbetts
The bibliography (with holdings) of printed maps of the Arabian Peninsula from attempts based on Ptolemy to the modern period. With many illustrations in colour and monochrome.

ALBANIA: A TRAVEL GUIDE
Philip Ward
What should the 1980s visitor look for in isolated Marxist Albania, known as Tibet-in-Europe? The author records a journey from Shkodër to Butrint and back. Copiously illustrated.

ROSSYA: A JOURNEY THROUGH SIBERIA
Michael Pennington
The Royal Shakespeare Company actor's chronicle of the crossing of Siberia by rail, with a stop-off at Irkutsk. Illustrated by the actor Roger Rees.

THE AEOLIAN ISLANDS
Philip Ward
Stromboli, Lipari and Vulcano are the best-known of the Aeolian archipelago north of Sicily. But other islands are unspoilt and each is unique in its own way.